ANTI-INFLAMMATORY DIET

4-Week Meal Plan for Beginners with Easy Recipes to Fight Inflammation and Restore Your Healthy Weight

Emma Green

Copyright © 2018 by Emma Green.

All rights reserved.

No part of this book may be reproduced in any form or by any electronic or mechanical means – except in the case of brief quotation embodied in articles or reviews – without written permission from its publisher.

Disclaimer

The recipes and information in this book are provided for educational purposes only. Please always consult a licensed professional before making changes to your lifestyle or diet. The author and/or publisher shall have neither liability nor responsibility to anyone with respect to any loss or damage caused or alleged to be caused directly or indirectly by the information contained in this book. All trademarks and brands within this book are for clarifying purposes only and are owned by the owners themselves, not affiliated with this document.

Images from shutterstock.com

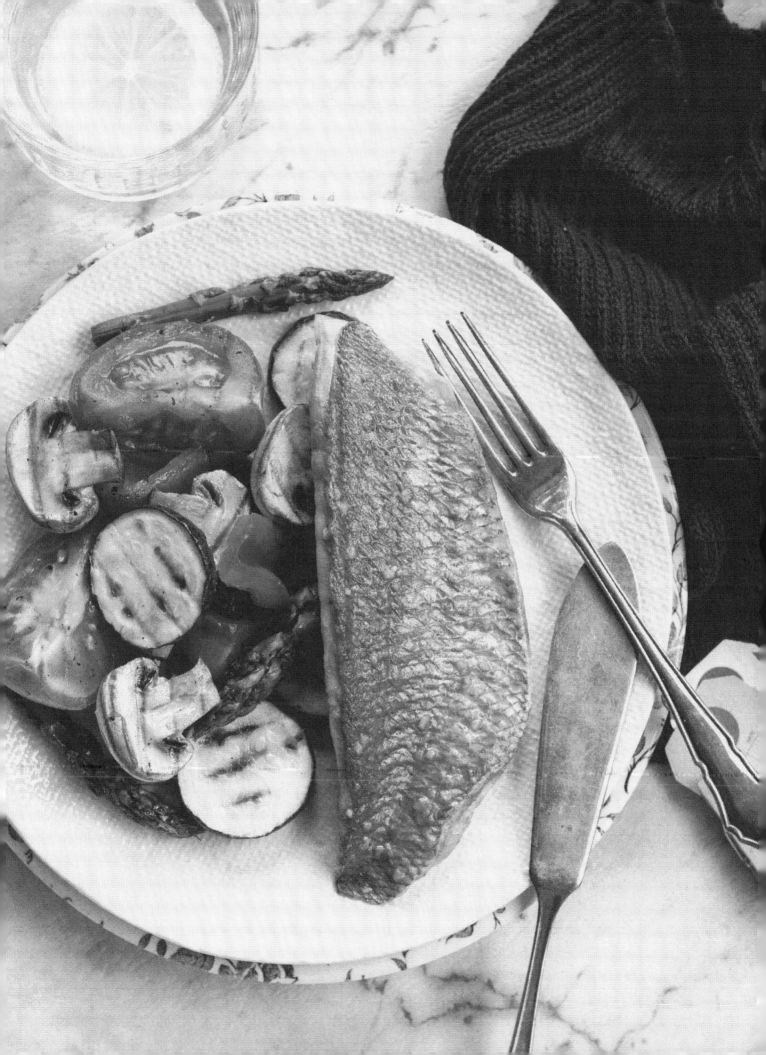

CONTENTS

INTRODUCTION 6

CHAPTER 1. The Basics 7
- Understanding Inflammation 7
- What is the Anti-inflammatory Diet 8
- What to Avoid on the Anti-inflammatory Diet 10
- What to Eat on the Anti-inflammation Diet 13
- Common Misconceptions about the Anti-inflammatory Diet 16

CHAPTER 2. Four-Week Anti-inflammation Meal Plan 17

CHAPTER 3. Recipes 21

BREAKFAST 21
- Avocado and Egg Toast 21
- Lemony Chia Quinoa Bowl 22
- Chia Breakfast Pudding 23
- Coconut Rice with Berries 24
- Overnight Muesli 25
- Spicy Quinoa 26
- Buckwheat Crêpes with Berries 27
- Mushroom "Frittata" 28

SNACKS 29
- Cucumber-Yogurt Dip 29
- Mashed Avocado with Jicama Slices 30
- Smoked Trout & Mango Wraps 31
- Smoked Turkey–Wrapped Zucchini Sticks 32
- Sweet Potato Chips 33
- Mini Snack Muffins 34
- Plantain Fries with Garlic & Rosemary 35
- Oven-Roasted Parsnips 36

SOUPS & STEWS 37
- Tuscan White Beans Stew 37
- Broccoli & Lentil Stew 38
- Mango & Black Bean Stew 39
- Coconut Fish Stew 40
- Roasted Vegetable Soup 41
- Mushrooms in Broth 42
- Fennel, Leek & Pear Soup 43
- Lentil & Carrot Soup with Ginger 44

SALADS 45
- Avocado & Grapefruit Salad 45
- Super Pineapple Almond Salad 46
- Brussels Sprout Slaw 47
- Quinoa and Roasted Asparagus Salad 48
- White Bean & Tuna Salad 49

- Mango Salsa 50
- Mediterranean Chopped Salad 51

MAIN DISHES 52
- Trout with Sweet-and-Sour Chard 52
- Pecan-Crusted Trout 53
- Sea Bass Baked with Tomatoes, Olives & Capers 54
- Swordfish with Pineapple & Cilantro 55
- Chicken Breast with Cherry Sauce 56
- Cheesy Cauliflower 57
- Immune-Boosting Rice Congee 58
- Chicken with Brown Rice & Snow Peas 59
- Chicken Thighs with Sweet Potatoes 60

SIDE DISHES 61
- Spicy Cauliflower 61
- Strawberry Avocado Tostada 62
- Rosemary Squash 63
- Scrumptious Green Beans 64
- Simple & Delectable Beets 65
- Cauliflower Purée 66
- Green Beans with Crispy Shallots 67

DESSERTS 68
- Banana-Cocoa Ice 68
- Melon with Berry-Yogurt Sauce 69
- Cherry "Ice Cream" 70
- Chocolate-Avocado Mousse with Sea Salt 71
- Chocolate-Cherry Clusters 72
- Baked Red Apples 73
- Coconut Vanilla "Ice Cream" 74
- Mochi with Yogurt 75

SMOOTHIES & DRINKS 76
- Inflammation-Soothing Smoothie 76
- Cherry Smoothie 77
- Eat-Your-Vegetables Smoothie 78
- Green Apple Smoothie 79
- One-for-All Smoothie 80
- Mango-Thyme Smoothie 81
- Protein Powerhouse Smoothie 82
- Energizing Pineapple Breakfast Smoothie 83

Recipe Index 84
Conversion Tables 85
Other Books by Emma Green 86

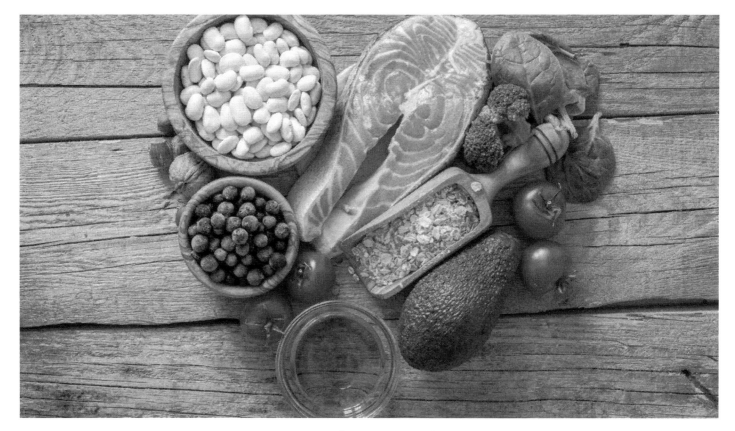

INTRODUCTION

Many people consider inflammation an attack on their body. The truth, however, is that inflammation is a natural process your body uses to protect itself. Usually, inflammation is a result of a number of chemical reactions caused by your body's hormones to fight infections or rebalance body chemicals. Inflammation and pain are simply signs that there is something wrong with our bodies. This could be an attack by pathogens, nutritional deficiency or excess accumulation of certain nutrients. Research has linked body inflammation to a number of medical conditions such as diabetes, cancer, heart diseases, chronic obstructive lung diseases, and Alzheimer's disease among others.

Research shows that a lot of things can, on the other hand, help reduce and cure inflammation. These include reducing your stress levels, exercising regularly and choosing what you eat. What we eat has a lot of influence on how our bodies react. This is because our bodies are built by the food we eat and eating the right kind of food can help reduce a lot of health-related complications that are associated with inflammation.

Eating certain diets can help decrease inflammation and other disease symptoms. Diets that help reduce inflammation are generally referred to as anti-inflammatory diets. These diets are made of specially selected foods that help supply your body's nutrients while providing soothing chemicals to help reduce inflammations.

This book offers a step-by-step approach to changing your nutrition and even your lifestyle habits. Detailed information will help you to get closer to your goal with every step you take. Good luck!

CHAPTER 1. The Basics

Understanding Inflammation

Nowadays inflammation has become one of the greatest interests of medical research. Barely a week goes by without another study reporting a new way chronic inflammation does harm to the body. Now we can claim that chronic inflammation may be the engine that drives most of the feared illnesses of middle and old age.

To make it clear, inflammation, nevertheless, is a natural response to trauma, infection, disease, and other physical assaults. It helps to rid the body of bacteria and toxins. It also "mops up" dead cells and tissues. Without inflammation, injured tissues would not heal, and infections would flame out of control.

However, chronic inflammation is not a good response. It's a long inflammatory immune response that eventually leads to tissue damage. It's low grade and systemic. It can provoke a domino effect that causes serious damage to your health. Generally, it is the root of many illnesses mainly because of poor diet, allergic reactions, stress, toxins, or psychological issues.

One of the most destructive inflammatory molecules is called nuclear factor kappa B. It is a small molecule that creates significant damage to the body. Emotional stress; toxic, inflammatory, or allergenic foods; and free radicals can activate it. When it is set off, it can unleash the production of numerous inflammatory molecules which might show up in a finger joint, your knees, your arteries, or your heart.

It is considered that more than half of all Americans have inflammation and most of them don't even know it. Many ailments are associated with chronic inflammation, including lupus, rheumatoid arthritis, fibromyalgia, atherosclerosis, inflammatory bowel disease, chronic pancreatitis, and chronic hepatitis among others. New research also links obesity with inflammation. Being overweight promotes inflammation and inflammation promotes obesity—a continuous and frustrating cycle.

Our bodies weren't designed for a daily barrage of toxins, infectious agents, genetically modified food, pesticide-sprayed food, refined foods, or intense, prolonged stress. This kind of demand requires significant support to maintain the immune system's resilience. Our on-the-go lifestyle doesn't tend toward immune support unless we pay particular attention to everything we do—what we breathe, eat, drink, think, and feel.

While the incidence of inflammation and inflammatory disease is increasing in all developed countries, we have a choice in how we respond to the causes of stress in our lives, along with what we choose to eat and drink, and how we think. There are many things in life that are beyond our control, but if you're lucky, your diet is not one of them. It's important to know about foods that worsen inflammation, the best anti-inflammatory fare to include in your diet, and how you can follow an anti-inflammatory diet. With this information, you can make smart choices at the grocery store to fuel and enhance a healthy lifestyle.

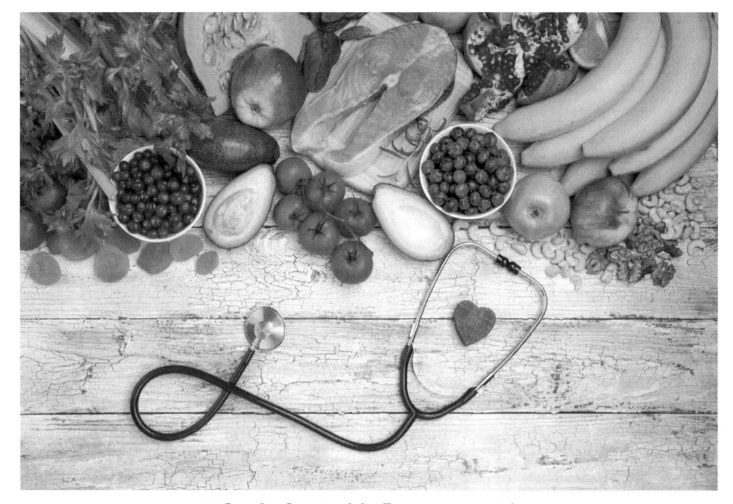

What is the Anti-inflammatory Diet

Food is a part of the solution to inflammation and to bringing your body under control. You may cool the inflammation fire with the right eating plan and recipes. An anti-inflammatory diet involves substituting sugary, refined foods with whole, nutrient-rich foods. It also contains increased amounts of antioxidants, which are reactive molecules in food that reduce the number of free radicals. Free radicals are molecules that may cause damage to cells in the body and increase the risk of certain diseases.

The Anti-inflammatory Diet is not a diet in the typical understanding — it is not intended as a weight-loss eating regimen (although people can and do lose weight on it), nor a diet to stay on for a limited period of time. It is rather, a way of choosing and preparing anti-inflammatory foods based on scientific knowledge of how they can help your body maintain health. This natural anti-inflammatory diet will provide steady energy and ample vitamins, minerals, essential fatty acids, dietary fiber, and protective phytonutrients.

General anti-inflammatory diet principles:

- Try to eat only organically grown foods to decrease your exposure to pesticides. Reduce the number of food additives and colorings, and increase the number of beneficial vitamins, minerals, and antioxidants consumed, which are used by the body to fight cancer and chronic disease.
- There is no preset restriction on the amount of food you can eat, and there is no need to count calories.
- Pay attention to your body's own satiety signals.
- Eat when you're hungry, and stop eating when you're satisfied.
- The specific foods listed below are only examples of foods to eat, so experiment.

- Try to plan meals with approximately the following caloric composition: 40 percent carbohydrates, 30 percent protein, and 30 percent healthy fats.
- Do not eat any one food more than five times per week.
- Plan your meals ahead of time.

Your lifestyle habits also matter when you want to gain as many benefits from the diet as possible. Our current home and work habits often fail to allow for a regular meal schedule. People's busy lives may prevent their caloric intake from being evenly distributed throughout the day.

Here are my suggestions for enhancing the quality of mealtimes:
- Spend time with your food. Do not do anything else such as watching TV, driving, or talking on the phone. Have a quiet, relaxed atmosphere in which to enjoy your food. Reflect upon the energy the food holds and what it is giving to you. Do not drink anything while eating. If you must have something, it should be limited to small sips of water.
- Proper chewing is an important part of digestion and should be something that you concentrate on during each meal. If you fail to chew your food thoroughly, digestion is not properly initiated, and your body will less adequately absorb important nutrients. I suggest that people chew their food at least nineteen times before swallowing.
- It is best to eat your meals at regularly scheduled times. Eating at the same times each day will establish a pattern with your endocrine system, helping to facilitate digestion at those times. Do not eat late at night, when your metabolism is getting ready to rest.
- Make sure to eat breakfast. Eating a whole-grain breakfast has been related to a 15 percent reduction in the risk of insulin resistance, a condition that can lead to type-II diabetes, weight gain, and cardiovascular complications. Refined "kid's" cereals, bread, pastries, and other carbohydrates typically consumed for breakfast will not have the same effect as whole grains. Eating all meals, starting with breakfast, is important to maintaining a revved-up metabolism throughout the day.

The cooking process and the fact of getting pleasure from what you are doing also plays a great role. So experiment and be creative. You can use many of the recipes in this book as a template for even greater meals. If you lack one or two ingredients, replace them with something you do have. I have included some simple beginning recipes that can go in many different directions. Don't be afraid to mix vegetables or grains with fruit. Adding a small amount of fruit to a green salad can be a refreshing treat on a summer day. Experiment with herbs and spices. Each week, choose one new seasoning to play with and learn about. Look up its medicinal properties, and be appreciative of its actions in your body. Cook to please yourself and, of course, anyone else dining with you.

Cooking healthily can take very little time. Although it is a passion of mine to spend hours in the kitchen cutting vegetables and preparing meals, I also have a busy health-care practice, a husband, and a child to tend to. I am no stranger to "quick meals." Thinking ahead of time helps to make even quick meals nutritious and full of life-giving energy. One time-saving hint is to chop vegetables ahead of time—for example, when you get home from the grocery store. If I know that I will be preparing a few different meals that require chopped onion, I will chop two to three onions and store them in an airtight container until I need them.

As with anything, the more you practice, the better cook you will become. Host weekly or monthly potlucks with friends and family to share and learn recipes. Most of my inspiration for cooking has come from my fellow naturopathic colleagues, including my husband. It is important to have support when changing your diet. Get your family members and friends involved, and most of all, have fun.

So, let's make clear what you should and should not eat when on an anti-inflammatory diet.

What to Avoid on the Anti-inflammatory Diet

Food choices can either soothe inflammation or cause it to worsen. This section details the foods that should be avoided on an anti-inflammatory diet.

Gluten

Gluten is a protein found in wheat, wheat germ, barley, rye, spelt, kamut, farro, bulgur, semolina, farina, and triticale. As gluten is hard to digest it can cause intestinal and digestive problems. But gluten causes more than digestive distress—it can also be responsible for brain fog, sinus problems, joint pain, blood sugar imbalances, hormonal imbalances, and skin conditions.

Despite media reports that gluten-free diets are only necessary for those with celiac disease, gluten consumption can worsen a wide range of chronic diseases. Anyone with virtually any inflammatory condition can benefit from a gluten-free diet.

The key principle of a healthy gluten-free diet is focusing on fresh, whole, naturally gluten-free foods. Skip the gluten with gluten-free grains, beans, legumes, nuts, seeds, lean meat, and fish instead. A diet rich in these foods will provide the nutrients you need to thrive and leave you feeling satisfied.

Gluten is often used as a binder or thickener in foods and, as such, that food can be a hidden source of it. Read food labels carefully and know these primary sources to check for gluten:

- Beer
- Bread
- Bread crumbs
- Cakes
- Candy
- Cereal
- Cookies
- Croutons
- Dairy
- Deli meats
- Flour
- Gravies
- Pasta and noodles
- Pasta sauce
- Pastries
- Salad dressings
- Sauces
- Soups
- Soy sauce

Dairy

Children are taught that dairy is an essential food to grow big and strong. However, many people don't produce the lactase enzyme required to digest the lactose sugars in milk, leading to bloating, gas, and diarrhea. In addition to lactose intolerance, milk allergies are quite common and are one of the top allergies in North American children.

Milk is a mucus-forming food, and when that mucus coats the digestive tract, it prevents nutrients from being absorbed. Dairy cows raised for conventional milk products are fed growth hormones and antibiotics, which can interfere with our hormones and lead to inflammation. Additionally, conventional dairy products are often loaded with sugar and preservatives (especially the low-fat ones), and this can further contribute to inflammatory processes.

While this information applies to many, it's good to note that some people may be able to eat dairy even though it's on the "foods to avoid" list.

Dairy foods to avoid:

- Butter
- Cheese
- Cottage cheese
- Cream cheese
- Frozen yogurt
- Ice cream
- Kefir
- Milk and cream
- Yogurt

Corn

Because so much corn today is genetically modified, it is food to avoid. About 90 percent of corn in the United States is genetically engineered. Genetically modified organisms (GMOs), or genetically modified foods, are relatively new to our food system and can pose potentially serious health risks. As a result of the modifications, they can suppress the immune system and promote inflammation. Corn is ubiquitous in processed foods; for instance, high-fructose corn syrup is prevalent in the majority of processed, sugary treats. And vegetable oils like corn oil are higher in omega-6 fatty acids, which are also inflammatory.

Try to avoid these foods:

- Corn
- Corn flour
- Corn oil
- Corn starch
- Corn sugar
- Corn syrup
- Corn tortillas
- Cornmeal
- Dextrin
- Dextrose
- Golden syrup
- High-fructose
- Maize
- Maltose
- Maltodextrin
- Xanthan gum

Soy

Similar to corn, this controversial bean is a common allergen. A recent report from the US Department of Agriculture's Economic Research Service states that 93 percent of soy grown in the United States is genetically modified. Soy is high in goitrogens—compounds that can suppress thyroid function. Soy also contains anti-nutrients such as phytates and oxalates, which interfere with digestion and disrupt the endocrine system.

Try to avoid these soy foods:

- Bean curd
- Edamame
- Miso
- Soybeans
- Soy flakes
- Soy flour
- Soy ice cream
- Soy isolate
- Soy lecithin
- Soy milk
- Soy nuts
- Soy oil
- Soy protein
- Peanuts
- Soy sauce
- Soy yogurt
- Tamari
- Tempeh
- Textured vegetable protein (TVP)
- Tofu

A common allergen, peanuts contain a carcinogenic mold called aflatoxin, which can affect those with liver conditions or candida. Peanut crops are heavily treated with pesticides, and this can lead to further inflammation or allergic reactions. They are also high in omega-6 fatty acids, a pro-inflammatory fat, and conventional peanut butter are loaded with added sugar and trans fats.

Caffeine

Can't survive without that morning caffeine jolt or afternoon pick-me-up? If you're suffering from inflammation, consider nixing your caffeine habit. Caffeine compels the stomach to release its contents prematurely, injecting undigested food into the small intestine, where it can aggravate the digestive tract. Caffeine sends blood sugar soaring, raises blood pressure and heart rate, suppresses appetite, and disrupts sleep. To put the final nail in the caffeine coffin, it stresses the nervous system, which can interfere with cortisol levels. Some practitioners recommend avoiding raw cocoa powder as well because cocoa (and any chocolate product) contains caffeine.

Alcohol

While the occasional glass of wine offers a positive hit of antioxidants, excess consumption of alcohol can increase the production of C-reactive protein (CRP), a marker of inflammation. Many alcoholic beverages are loaded with sugar, which can wreak havoc on blood sugar levels, cause headaches, and suppress the immune system. Alcohol also destroys gut flora, an integral part of the digestive system. Poor intestinal flora can lead to a leaky gut, where particles of food break through the intestinal barrier and activate the immune system, inducing further inflammation and allergies.

Citrus Foods

Most citrus foods are acidic and can provoke inflammation in people with conditions such as gastroesophageal reflux disease (GERD), arthritis, and citrus sensitivities. To buffer the acidity, the body pulls from its pool of alkaline minerals such as calcium, magnesium, and potassium. Without this buffer, the acid can place undue stress on the body, leaving one susceptible to disease. When used in moderation, though, lemons and limes can be a handy addition to an anti-inflammatory diet as they kick-start digestion and enhance liver detoxification. Once metabolized by the body, they leave alkaline minerals behind. Some other types of citrus also contain beneficial antioxidants and anti-inflammatory nutrients and can be helpful if consumed sparingly. Overall, however, it is better to avoid them.

Citrus foods to limit or avoid:

- Clementines
- Grapefruit
- Lemons
- Limes
- Oranges
- Pomelos
- Tangelos
- Tangerines
- Satsumas

Feedlot Animal Products

Conventional animal products from large, industrial animal farms—the biggest producers of meat in the US—cause inflammation for a variety of reasons. Animals are fed hormones and antibiotics. The latter have caused a growing worldwide problem of antibiotic resistance. Animals are often fed fare that is different from their natural diet. In feedlots, animals are mostly given grains like wheat and GMO corn, along with GMO soy—all of which are pro-inflammatory. Grain-fed animals also yield meat that is higher in inflammatory omega-6 fatty acids. As the old adage says, "Garbage in, garbage out." But you

can avoid this dilemma. Choose organic products from animals raised without hormones or antibiotics, with outdoor access, and fed a mix of grass and grain. If you don't have access to organic meat, check with your local farmer—sometimes farms follow organic practices, but cannot afford to become certified organic (it's very expensive to do so). Simply ask! You may find it's easier to access naturally raised meats and dairy than you thought.

Feedlot animal foods to avoid:

- Beef
- Broth
- Chicken
- Dairy
- Eggs
- Gelatin
- Goat
- Lamb, non-organic
- Pork
- Sheep
- Turkey

Artificial or Processed Foods

Processed foods contain many ingredients that contribute to inflammation: chemicals, preservatives, unhealthy fats, excess sugars, additives, artificial food dyes, refined carbohydrates, and synthetic vitamins and minerals the body cannot process, and more. As a general rule, if there is an ingredient on a food label that you can't make at home or that you won't find in nature, the best practice is to leave the product on the shelf.

Eggs

According to Health Canada, eggs are a top allergen in North America and can be difficult to digest, and many people are sensitive or intolerant to their protein. Feedlot eggs are particularly high in inflammatory nutrients, such as omega-6 fatty acids. While this information applies to many, it's good to note that some people may be able to eat eggs even though they're on the "foods to avoid" list. For more information on why this is the case, refer to Foods with Sensitivity Alerts. And on the flip side, organic pastured eggs are a great source of protein, vitamin D, omega-3 fatty acids, and B vitamins—especially choline, which is essential to the nervous system.

Nightshade Vegetables

This family of vegetables includes tomatoes, white potatoes, eggplant, peppers, and also tobacco. Nightshades contain alkaloids that can cause gastrointestinal upset, and may aggravate inflammation in conditions like rheumatoid arthritis and osteoarthritis, headaches, lupus, kidney disease, gout, hypertension, and cancer. Nightshade foods may also leach calcium from bones and redistribute it to places where it shouldn't be, like joints, kidneys, and arteries. And, again, while this information applies to many, it's good to note that some people may be able to eat vegetables in the nightshade family even though they're on the "foods to avoid" list.

What to Eat on the Anti-inflammation Diet

The good news: After reading about which foods to avoid, it might seem there's nothing left to eat. Not true. There is an abundance of foods you can enjoy, and the recipes in this book show you how to prepare them deliciously. You won't feel deprived in the least! Generally speaking, vegetables and fruits are your anti-inflammatory best friends. The following foods and food groups are packed with nutrients that prevent or reduce inflammation. Eat up!

Allium vegetables

Onions, garlic, leeks, shallots, scallions, ramps, and chives offer a host of benefits. Onions are a rich source of vitamin C and quercetin (which helps relieve allergy symptoms). Garlic is no slouch either; it contains a range of sulfurous compounds that reduce inflammation throughout the body, plus it has antiviral and antibacterial properties.

Basil

Eugenol, a volatile oil found in basil, inhibits the enzymes that produce inflammation (and actually effects the same enzymes targeted by NSAIDs).

Berries

Blueberries, raspberries, blackberries, and strawberries are potent sources of antioxidants that combat cellular damage and inhibit the enzymes that promote inflammation. Berries are also high in fiber, which benefits the digestive tract, cardiovascular system, and blood sugar levels.

Bone broth

Bone broth, prepared with organic animal bones, simmered for at least several hours, contains the amino acids glycine, proline, and arginine. It helps support the digestive tract by bringing digestive juices to the gut, and also reduces joint pain.

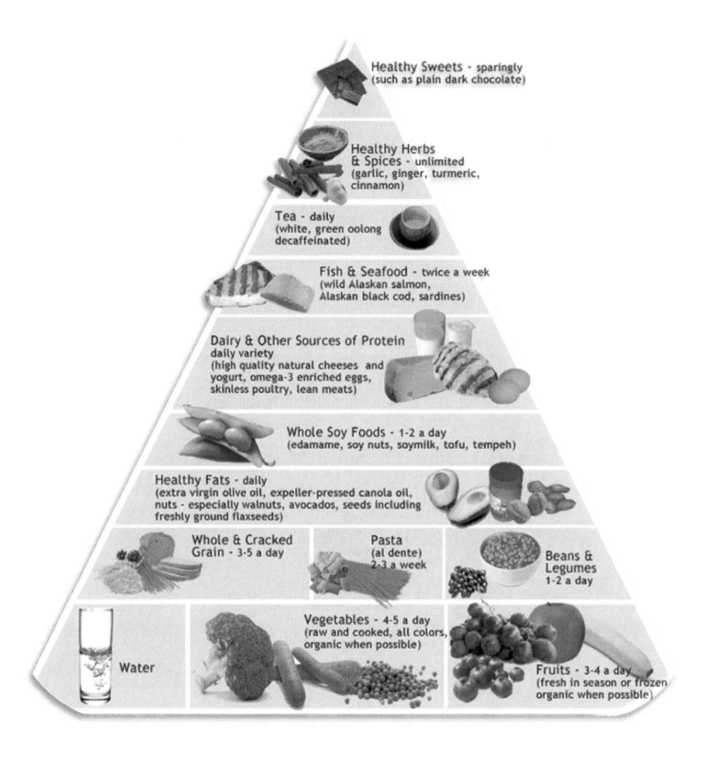

Coconut oil and extra-virgin olive oil

Coconut oil is a healthy saturated fat that is especially high in lauric acid, which enhances brain function and the immune system. It is easily digested and used immediately by the body for energy rather than being stored as fat. The extra-virgin olive oil contains numerous polyphenols that reduce the chemical messengers and enzymes that lead to inflammation.

Dark leafy greens

Dark leafy greens contain the antioxidant vitamins A, C, E, and K, which combat cellular damage that can contribute to inflammation. They're also great sources of anti-inflammatory omega-3 fatty acids and B vitamins, which help manage stress and nourish the nervous system.

Dill

This herb helps neutralize carcinogens and is used for digestive problems like gas, indigestion, and constipation.

Fennel

This sweet vegetable decreases processes that trigger inflammation. Fennel also contains antioxidants and immune-boosting nutrients

Fish

Wild salmon, sardines, anchovies, mackerel, and halibut are wonderful sources of omega-3 fatty acids—the healthy fats. Salmon, in particular, is high in two omega-3s called EPA and DHA, which help produce anti-inflammatory molecules.

Ginger

This root contains anti-inflammatory compounds called gingerols, which inhibit pro-inflammatory molecules. Ginger is used to treating a wide variety of conditions, including digestive issues, nausea, motion sickness, arthritis, headaches, colds, and flu

Gluten-free grains

Quinoa and brown rice are used throughout the anti-inflammatory recipes here and for a good reason. Quinoa is a complete plant-based source of protein, which means it has the same amino acids found in animal products. Sufficient protein is key to healing inflammation. It's also a rich source of magnesium, a relaxant mineral that reduces inflammation, and contains vitamin E. Brown rice is also high in magnesium as well as selenium, which helps with detoxification and protects cells from damage.

Natural sweeteners

While refined white sugars are inflammatory, there are some natural sweeteners that can be used in an anti-inflammatory diet. Raw honey is rich in healing amino acids, digestive enzymes, and antiviral constituents—helping to enhance the immune system. Maple syrup is rich in antioxidants, plus it's high in zinc—another important nutrient for the immune system. Of course, using natural sugars is completely optional. Omit them if you prefer to avoid sweeteners completely.

Nuts and seeds

Walnuts, almonds, cashews, hemp seeds, chia seeds, flaxseed, and more contain a wide range of healthy fats, protein, and fiber. Walnuts, hemp seed, chia seeds, and flax seed are particularly high in omega-3 fatty acids.

Pineapple

The core and stem of this tropical fruit contain bromelain, which reduces inflammation and helps protein digestion.

Root vegetables

Carrots, sweet potatoes, parsnips, turnips, celery root, rutabaga, and beets are anti-inflammatory and antioxidant powerhouses. Carrots and sweet potatoes are rich sources of vitamin A, which helps nourish the mucosal cells in the digestive tract, aids vision, boosts the immune system and keeps skin healthy. Sweet potatoes contain anthocyanin pigments and beets are full of compounds called betalains, both of which reduce the production of inflammatory enzymes.

Sustainable, organic meat

Lamb, chicken, and turkey are high in protein, which is essential for healing and repairing inflammation. They are also rich in B vitamins, particularly B12—a key nutrient for the nervous system rarely present in plants.

Turmeric

Turmeric's anti-inflammatory power stems from curcumin. It can help reduce the inflammation associated with inflammatory bowel disease, arthritis, cystic fibrosis, and cancer.

Winter squashes

Similar to root vegetables, winter squashes contain high amounts of vitamins C and A. They also contain special compounds called cucurbitacins that inhibit the enzymes that lead to inflammation.

Common Misconceptions about the Anti-inflammatory Diet

There is no exact definition of an anti-inflammatory diet, and the definition depends on whom you ask. Consequently, there are a lot of misconceptions about this diet. Let`s clarify some myths for you to get rid of, and instead focus on what really matters to boost your health. Some of the major misunderstanding and mistakes about the anti-inflammatory diet are as follows:

- **"An anti-inflammatory diet is a restrictive diet"**

People are trying to control their eating for one reason or another often end up with very strict diets. They create a list of foods to avoid and end up with joyless diets that may also compromise their nutritional intake. Sometimes, the very restrictive diets may even cause more health problems than they help. The truth of the matter is that anti-inflammatory diets are made up of a wide variety of foods and only work on limiting the amount of intake as opposed to the elimination of foods from your diets. This ensures you enjoy tasty meals in the right quantities without having to think too much about restricting foods.

- **"Spicy foods cause inflammation"**

This misconception comes from the middle ages. Many people believe that spicy foods are the cause of many health problems. The truth is some spices may worsen certain medical conditions, but there is not any scientific proof that spices cause diseases. So as you plan your anti-inflammatory diets ensure that you consider each food substance to be included as opposed to following such generalizations.

- **"There is a one-fits-all recipe when it comes to anti-inflammatory diets"**

This is another misconception about the ability of many people to use anti-inflammatory diets. The truth is different people suffer from different kinds of inflammation caused by different agents. So, what works for one person may not work in a similar manner for another person. There are many conditions involved when it comes to inflammation, and this can affect how your body reacts to certain foods. It is very important to take this fact into account and experiment with various foods until you find what works for you. If you try a certain diet and find out that it does not work for you, don't just give up on the whole issue but try out other different meals to see if they work for you.

- **"Milk causes inflammation"**

There are a lot of reports that suggest that milk is bad for our health. However, studies have shown that milk and other dairy products have anti-inflammatory properties and can actually protect from chronic inflammation.

CHAPTER 2. Four-Week Anti-inflammation Meal Plan

A diet high in plant-based protein, complex carbohydrates, fiber, and healthy fats, this "action plan" is great for vegetarians or vegans. If you want to increase your plant consumption and explore plant-based recipes, this is a great way to start. However, for anyone who cannot tolerate beans, legumes, or grains, this is not the plan for you. Likewise, meat lovers be forewarned: you may not be fully satisfied.

Week 1

	Breakfast	Lunch	Snack	Dinner
Monday	Inflammation-Soothing Smoothie Page 76	Fennel, Leek, and Pear Soup Page 43	Celery and ¼ cup of almond butter	Trout with Sweet-and-Sour Chard Page 52
Tuesday	Avocado and Egg Toast Page 21	Brussels Sprout Slaw Page 47	Fruit and 8 ounces plain nondairy yogurt	Tuscan White Beans Stew Page 37
Wednesday	Eat-Your-Vegetables Smoothie Page 78	Fennel, Leek, and Pear Soup (leftovers) Page 43	Smoked Trout & Mango Wraps Page 31	Pecan-Crusted Trout Page 53
Thursday	Coconut Rice with Berries Page 24	Mushrooms in Broth Page 42	Mini-snack Muffins Page 34	Immune-Boosting Rice Congee Page 58
Friday	Protein Powerhouse Smoothie Page 82	Lentil & Carrot Soup with Ginger Page 44	Apple and ½ cup of almonds	Sea Bass Baked with Tomatoes, Olives & Capers Page 54
Saturday	Chia Breakfast Pudding Page 23	Lentil & Carrot Soup with Ginger (leftovers) Page 44	Half an avocado sprinkled with sea salt	Broccoli & Lentil Stew Page 38
Sunday	Buckwheat Crêpes with Berries Page 27	Roasted Vegetable Soup Page 41	Mashed Avocado with Jicama Slices Page 30	Swordfish with Pineapple & Cilantro Page 55

Week 2

	Breakfast	Lunch	Snack	Dinner
Monday	One-for-All Smoothie Page 80	Avocado & Grapefruit Salad Page 45	Plantain Fries with Garlic & Rosemary Page 35	Coconut Fish Stew Page 40
Tuesday	Spicy Quinoa Page 26	Mango Salsa Page 50	Oven-Roasted Parsnips Page 36	Chicken Breast with Cherry Sauce Page 56
Wednesday	Green Apple Smoothie Page 79	Rosemary Squash Page 63	Sweet Potato Chips Page 33	Sea Bass Baked with Tomatoes, Olives & Capers Page 54
Thursday	Green Apple Smoothie Page 79	Fennel, Leek & Pear Soup Page 43	Celery with ¼ cup of almond butter	Swordfish with Pineapple & Cilantro Page 55
Friday	Lemony Chia Quinoa Bowl Page 22	Fennel, Leek & Pear Soup (leftovers) Page 43	Mashed Avocado with Jicama Slices Page 30	Chicken with Brown Rice & Snow Peas Page 59
Saturday	Buckwheat Crêpes with Berries Page 27	Quinoa and Roasted Asparagus Salad Page 48	Mini-snack Muffins Page 34	Tuscan White Beans Stew Page 37
Sunday	Green Beans with Crispy Shallots Page 67	Lentil & Carrot Soup with Ginger Page 44	¼ cup Green Olive Tapenade, with cucumber slices	Pecan-Crusted Trout Page 53

Week 3

	Breakfast	Lunch	Snack	Dinner
Monday	Cherry Smoothie Page 77	Strawberry Avocado Tostada Page 62	Half an avocado with sea salt	Pecan-Crusted Trout Page (leftovers) Page 53
Tuesday	Protein Powerhouse Smoothie Page 82	Mango & Black Bean Stew Page 39	Celery and ¼ cup of almond butter	Sea Bass Baked with Tomatoes, Olives & Capers Page 54
Wednesday	Protein Powerhouse Smoothie Page 82	White Bean and Tuna Salad Page 49	Pear and ½ cup of almonds	Trout with Sweet-and-Sour Chard Page 52
Thursday	Mushroom "Frittata" Page 28	Quinoa and Roasted Asparagus Salad Page 48	Carrot sticks and ¼ cup of hummus	Swordfish with Pineapple & Cilantro Page 55
Friday	Green Beans with Crispy Shallots Page 67	Lentil & Carrot Soup with Ginger Page 44	¼ cup Green Olive Tapenade, with cucumber slices	Pecan-Crusted Trout Page 53
Saturday	Green Beans with Crispy Shallots (leftovers) Page 67	Strawberry Avocado Tostada Page 62	Melon with Berry-Yogurt Sauce Page 69	Coconut Fish Stew Page 40
Sunday	Inflammation-Soothing Smoothie Page 76	Simple & Delectable Beets Page 65	Mochi with Yogurt Page 75	Super Pineapple Almond Salad Page 46

Week 4

	Breakfast	Lunch	Snack	Dinner
Monday	Coconut Rice with Berries Page 24	Spicy Cauliflower Page 61	Mashed Avocado with Jicama Slices Page 30	Tuscan White Beans Stew Page 37
Tuesday	Energizing Pineapple Breakfast Smoothie Page 83	Spicy Cauliflower Page 61	Plantain Fries with Garlic & Rosemary Page 35	Immune-Boosting Rice Congee Page 58
Wednesday	Spicy Quinoa Page 26	Roasted Vegetable Soup Page 41	Celery and ¼ cup of hummus	Chicken Thighs with Sweet Potatoes Page 60
Thursday	Green Apple Smoothie Page 79	Super Pineapple Almond Salad Page 46	Endive leaves with ¼ cup of Green Olive Tapenade	Pecan-Crusted Trout Page 53
Friday	Lemony Chia Quinoa Bowl Page 22	Roasted Vegetable Soup Page 41	Chocolate-Avocado Mousse with Sea Salt Page 71	Chicken Thighs with Sweet Potatoes Page 60
Saturday	Cherry Smoothie Page 77	Rosemary Squash Page 63	Oven-Roasted Parsnips Page 36	Tuscan White Beans Stew Page 37
Sunday	Buckwheat Crêpes with Berries Page 27	Mediterranean Chopped Salad Page 51	Strawberry Avocado Tostada Page 62	Chicken Thighs with Sweet Potatoes Page 60

CHAPTER 3. Recipes
BREAKFAST

Avocado and Egg Toast

Prep time: 5 minutes

Cooking time: 8 minutes

Servings: 1

Nutrients per serving:

Carbohydrates – 14.9 g

Fat – 31 g

Protein – 8.7 g

Calories – 356

Ingredients:

- 1 slice gluten-free bread, toasted
- ½ avocado
- 1 egg, scrambled or poached
- 1½ tsp of ghee
- 1 handful of spinach
- 1 tsp red pepper flakes

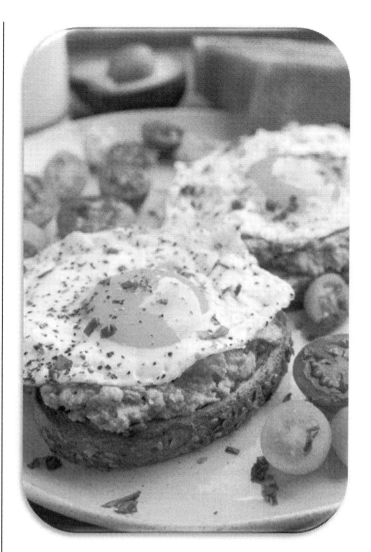

Instructions:

1. Toast the bread slice and top it with ghee.
2. Spread avocado on the toast. Place fresh leaves of spinach on top of avocado; then top everything with a scrambled or poached egg and finish it with a sprinkling of red pepper flakes. Serve.

Lemony Chia Quinoa Bowl

Prep time: 5 minutes

Cooking time: 15 minutes

Servings: 6

Nutrients per serving:

Carbohydrates – 38 g

Fat – 5 g

Protein – 5 g

Calories – 215

Ingredients:

- 1 cup of quinoa
- 1½ cups almond milk
- 3 tbsp slivered almonds
- 1 tbsp chia seeds
- 4½ tbsp pure maple syrup
- ¼ tsp sea salt
- 1 pinch of fresh lemon zest, grated

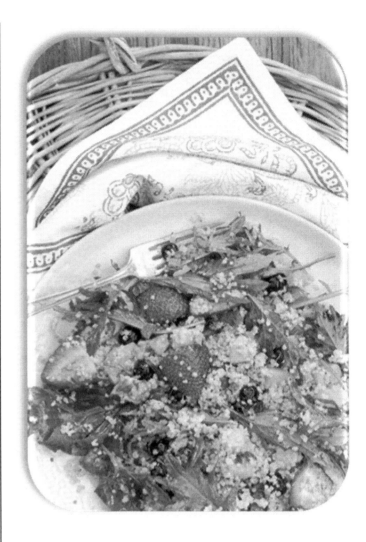

Instructions:

1. Cook the quinoa as per package directions.
2. Remove it from heat; keep aside for about 5 minutes and then fluff it with a fork and stir in almond milk, almonds, chia seeds, maple syrup, lemon zest and sea salt.
3. Mix well to combine and serve it warm.

Chia Breakfast Pudding

Prep time: 10 minutes (+15 minutes)

Cooking time: none

Servings: 4

Nutrients per serving:

Carbohydrates – 38 g

Fat – 14 g

Protein – 7 g

Calories – 272

Ingredients:

- 2 cups almond milk
- ½ cup chia seeds
- ¼ cup maple syrup or raw honey
- 1 tsp vanilla extract
- 1 cup frozen unsweetened pitted cherries, thawed, juice reserved, divided
- ½ cup chopped cashews, divided

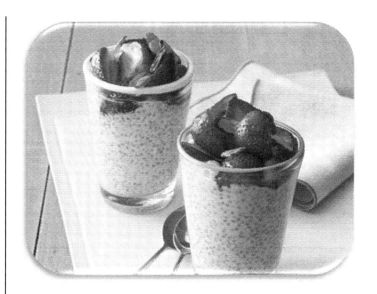

Instructions:

1. In a quart jar with a tight-fitting lid, combine the almond milk, chia seeds, maple syrup, and vanilla. Shake and set aside for at least 15 minutes. (You can also do this before bed and refrigerate overnight.)
2. Divide the pudding among four bowls, and top each with ¼ cup of cherries and 2 tbsp of cashews.

Coconut Rice with Berries

Prep time: 10 minutes

Cooking time: 30 minutes

Servings: 4

Nutrients per serving:

Carbohydrates – 49 g

Fat – 8 g

Protein – 6 g

Calories – 281

Ingredients:

- 1 cup brown basmati rice
- 1 cup water
- 1 cup coconut milk
- 1 tsp salt
- 2 dates, pitted, chopped
- 1 cup fresh blueberries, divided
- ¼ cup slivered almonds, toasted, divided
- ½ cup shaved coconut, divided

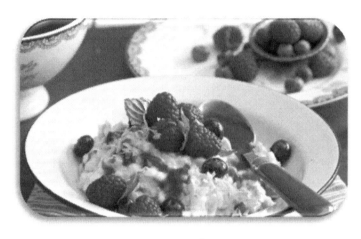

Instructions:

1. In a saucepan over high heat, combine the basmati rice, water, coconut milk, salt, and date pieces.
2. Bring the mixture to a boil. Reduce the heat to simmer and cook for 20 to 30 minutes, without stirring, or until the rice is tender.
3. Place the rice into four bowls and top each serving with ¼ cup of blueberries, 1 tbsp of almonds, and 2 tbsp of coconut.

Overnight Muesli

Prep time: 10 minutes (+8 hours)

Cooking time: none

Servings: 4–6

Nutrients per serving:

Carbohydrates – 39 g

Fat – 4 g

Protein – 6 g

Calories – 213

Ingredients:

- 2 cups gluten- free rolled oats
- 1¾ cups coconut milk
- ¼ cup unsweetened apple juice
- 1 apple, cored, chopped
- Dash ground cinnamon

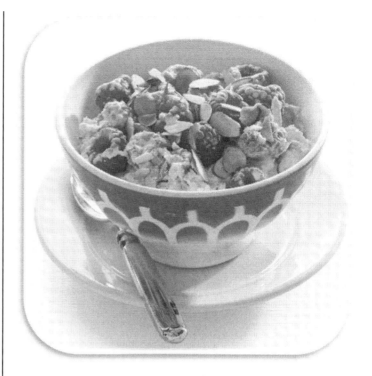

Instructions:

1. In a bowl, combine together the oats, coconut milk, and apple juice.
2. Cover and refrigerate overnight.
3. The next morning, stir in the chopped apple and season the muesli with the cinnamon.

Spicy Quinoa

Prep time: 10 minutes

Cooking time: 20 minutes

Servings: 4

Nutrients per serving:

Carbohydrates – 32 g

Fat – 13 g

Protein – 10 g

Calories – 286

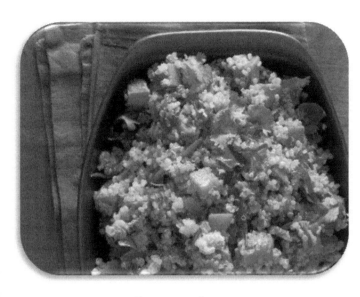

Ingredients:

- 1 cup quinoa, rinsed well
- 2 cups water
- ½ cup coconut, shredded
- ¼ cup hemp seeds
- 2 tbsp flaxseed
- 1 tsp cinnamon, ground
- 1 tsp vanilla extract
- Salt to taste
- 1 cup fresh berries of your choice, divided
- ¼ cup hazelnuts, chopped

Instructions:

1. In a saucepan over high heat, combine the quinoa and water.
2. Bring to a boil, then simmer for 15–20 minutes.
3. Stir in the coconut, hemp seeds, flaxseed, cinnamon, vanilla, and salt.
4. Divide the quinoa among four bowls and top each serving with a ¼ cup of berries and 1 tbsp of hazelnuts.

Buckwheat Crêpes with Berries

Prep time: 15 minutes

Cooking time: 20 minutes

Servings: 4

Nutrients per serving:

Carbohydrates – 33 g

Fat – 11 g

Protein – 7 g

Calories – 242

Ingredients:

- 1 cup buckwheat flour
- ½ tsp salt
- 2 tbsp coconut oil
- 1½ cups almond milk or water
- 1 egg
- 1 tsp vanilla extract
- 3 cups fresh berries, divided
- 6 tbsp Chia Jam, divided

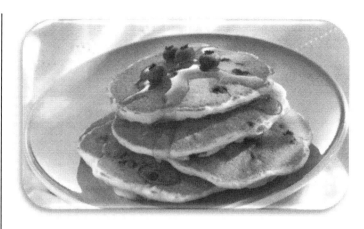

Instructions:

1. In a small bowl, whisk together the buckwheat flour, salt, 1 tbsp coconut oil, the almond milk or water, egg, and vanilla until smooth.
2. In a skillet, melt the remaining coconut oil. Tilt the pan, coating it evenly with the melted oil.
3. Ladle ¼ cup of batter into the skillet. Stir to coat with the batter.
4. Cook for 2 minutes. Flip the crêpe and cook for 1 minute on the second side. Transfer the crêpe to a plate.
5. Continue making crêpes with the remaining batter. You should have 4 to 6 crêpes.
6. Place 1 crêpe on a plate, top with ½ cup of berries and 1 tbsp of Chia Jam. Fold the crêpe over the filling. Repeat with the remaining crêpes and serve.

Mushroom "Frittata"

Prep time: 15 minutes

Cooking time: 35 minutes

Servings: 6

Nutrients per serving:

Carbohydrates – 34 g

Fat – 8 g

Protein – 11 g

Calories – 240

Ingredients:

- 1½ cups chickpea flour
- 1½ cups water
- 1 tsp salt
- 2 tbsp extra-virgin olive oil
- 1 small red onion, diced
- 2 pints mushrooms, sliced
- 1 tsp turmeric, ground
- ½ tsp cumin, ground
- Salt, pepper to taste
- 2 tbsp fresh parsley, chopped

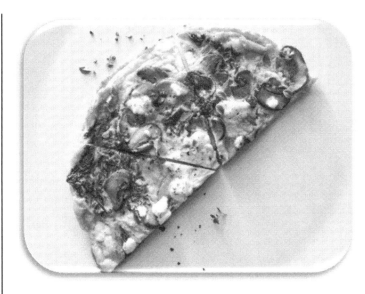

Instructions:

1. Preheat the oven to 350°F.
1. In a bowl, whisk the water into the chickpea flour; add the salt and set aside.
2. In an oven-safe skillet, add the olive oil, then onion. Sauté for 3–5 minutes. Add the mushrooms and sauté for another 5 minutes. Stir in the turmeric, cumin, salt, and pepper, and sauté for 1 minute.
3. Pour the batter over the vegetables. Bake for 20-25 minutes. Sprinkle with the parsley. Serve warm.

SNACKS

Cucumber-Yogurt Dip

Prep time: 15 minutes

Cooking time: none

Servings: 4

Nutrients per serving:

Carbohydrates – 7 g

Fat – 9 g

Protein – 1 g

Calories – 104

Ingredients:

- 1 cucumber, peeled, shredded
- 1 cup plain coconut milk yogurt
- 1 garlic clove, minced
- 1 scallion, chopped
- 2 tbsp fresh dill, chopped
- 1 tsp salt
- 2 tbsp freshly squeezed lemon juice
- 2 tbsp extra-virgin olive oil

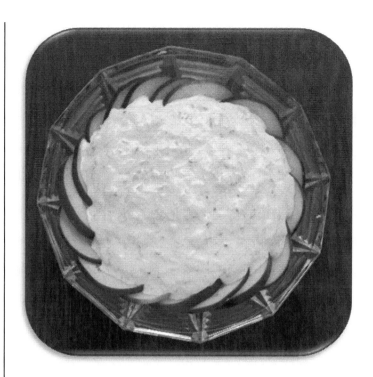

Instructions:

1. Place the shredded cucumber in a fine-mesh strainer to drain.
2. In a small bowl, stir together the yogurt, garlic, scallion, dill, salt, and lemon juice.
3. Fold in the drained cucumber and spoon into a serving bowl.
4. Drizzle with the olive oil, serve.

Mashed Avocado with Jicama Slices

Prep time: 15 minutes

Cooking time: none

Servings: 4

Nutrients per serving:

Carbohydrates – 24 g

Fat – 20 g

Protein – 3 g

Calories – 270

Ingredients:

- 2 ripe avocados, pitted
- 1 scallion, sliced
- 2 tbsp fresh cilantro, chopped
- ½ tsp turmeric, ground
- Salt, pepper to taste
- 1 jicama, peeled, sliced
- Juice of ½ lemon

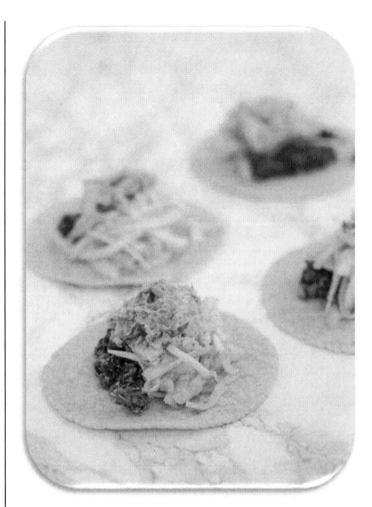

Instructions:

1. In a small bowl, combine the scooped-out avocado, the scallion, cilantro, turmeric, lemon juice, salt, and pepper. Mash the ingredients together until well mixed and still slightly chunky.
2. Serve with the jicama slices.

Smoked Trout & Mango Wraps

Prep time: 15 minutes

Cooking time: none

Servings: 4

Nutrients per serving:

Carbohydrates – 13 g

Fat – 3 g

Protein – 9 g

Calories – 108

Ingredients:

- 4 large green-leaf lettuce leaves, thick stems removed
- 4 ounces trout, smoked, divided
- 1 cup mango, chopped, divided
- 1 scallion, sliced, divided
- 2 tbsp lemon juice, freshly squeezed, divided

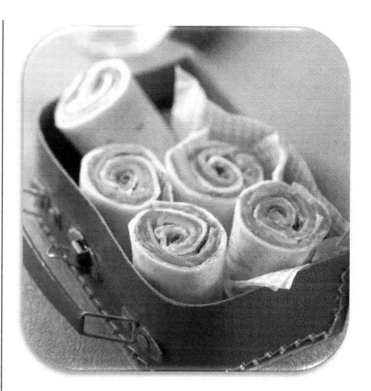

Instructions:

1. Place the lettuce leaves on a flat surface. Top each leaf equally with pieces of the trout and mango. Sprinkle with the scallions and drizzle with the lemon juice.
2. Wrap the lettuce leaves burrito style and place them seam-side down on a serving dish.

Smoked Turkey–Wrapped Zucchini Sticks

Prep time: 15 minutes

Cooking time: none

Servings: 4

Nutrients per serving:

Carbohydrates – 6 g

Fat – 3 g

Protein – 21 g

Calories – 137

Ingredients:

- 8 thin slices of turkey breast, smoked
- 2 zucchini, quartered lengthwise
- 1 cup packed arugula, divided
- Salt to taste

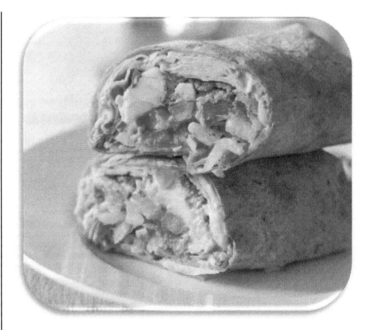

Instructions:

1. Place 1 slice of smoked turkey on a work surface. Top with 1 zucchini stick, ¼ cup of arugula, season with salt.
2. Wrap the turkey around the vegetables and place on a platter, seam-side down. Repeat with the remaining ingredients. Serve.

Sweet Potato Chips

Prep time: 20 minutes

Cooking time: 2 hours

Servings: 4

Nutrients per serving:

Carbohydrates – 42 g

Fat – 11 g

Protein – 2 g

Calories – 267

Ingredients:

- 2 large sweet potatoes, sliced
- 3 tbsp extra-virgin olive oil
- 1 tsp sea salt

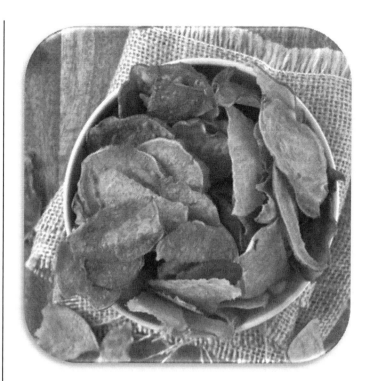

Instructions:

1. Preheat the oven to 250°F.
2. Put the rack in the center of the oven.
3. In a bowl, toss the sweet potatoes slices with the olive oil. Arrange the slices in a single layer on two baking sheets. Season with sea salt.
4. Place the sheets in the preheated oven and bake for about 2 hours, rotating the pans and flipping the chips after 1 hour.
5. Cool the chips for 10 minutes before serving.

Mini Snack Muffins

Prep time: 20 minutes

Cooking time: 20 minutes

Servings: 24

Nutrients per serving:

Carbohydrates – 7 g

Fat – 4 g

Protein – 2 g

Calories – 65

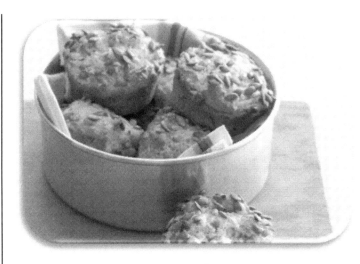

Ingredients:

- ¼ cup extra- virgin olive oil
- 1 cup almond flour
- 1 cup brown rice flour
- 1 tbsp baking powder
- ½ tsp salt
- 1 tsp cinnamon, ground
- 4 eggs
- 1 cup carrots, shredded
- 1 cup pumpkin, canned

Instructions:

1. Preheat the oven to 375°F.
2. Brush a mini-muffin tin with a little olive oil.
3. In a bowl, mix the almond flour, brown rice flour, baking powder, salt, and cinnamon.
4. Add the eggs, carrot, pumpkin, and olive oil. Stir until well combined.
5. Scoop the batter into muffin cups, filling each three-quarters full.
6. Bake for 15 minutes. Let chill before serving.

Plantain Fries with Garlic & Rosemary

Prep time: 10 minutes

Cooking time: 15 minutes

Servings: 3

Nutrients per serving:

Carbohydrates – 41 g

Fat – 10 g

Protein – 2.1 g

Calories – 241

Ingredients:

- 2 green plantains
- 2 tbsp olive oil
- 1 tbsp dried rosemary
- 1 tsp sea salt
- 8 garlic cloves, minced

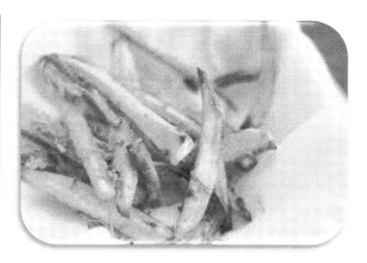

Instructions:

1. Preheat the oven to 425°F.
2. Peel the plantains and cut into strips.
3. In a mixing bowl, toss plantains in oil and mix with rosemary and sea salt. Put aluminum foil on a baking pan and spread fries in the pan.
4. Sprinkle minced garlic over the fries; bake them for 10 minutes. Remove the baking pan and rotate fries and bake for another 5 minutes.

Oven-Roasted Parsnips

Prep time: 10 minutes

Cooking time: 25 minutes

Servings: 4

Nutrients per serving:

Carbohydrates – 20 g

Fat – 4 g

Protein – 1.5 g

Calories – 110

Ingredients:

- 2 lb parsnips
- 1 tbsp extra-virgin olive oil
- 1 tsp kosher salt
- 1½ tsp of Herbs de Provence, or Italian seasoning
- Chopped parsley to taste

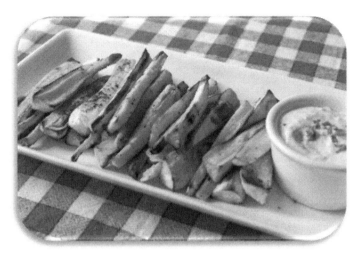

Instructions:

1. Preheat the oven to 400° F.
2. Peel the parsnips and cut them into chunks. Toss them with oil, salt, and herbs in a bowl. Spread them on an oiled baking sheet.
3. Roast for about 25–30 minutes. Stir a couple of times during roasting. Place them on a serving platter and top with parsley.

SOUPS & STEWS

Tuscan White Beans Stew

Prep time: 10 minutes

Cooking time: 35 minutes

Servings: 4

Nutrients per serving:

Carbohydrates – 3.2 g

Fat – 4.2 g

Protein – 2.8 g

Calories – 61

Ingredients:

- 1 can (15 oz) organic white beans
- 1 garlic clove
- ¼ cup onion
- ½ cup carrots
- 1/3 cup celery
- 1 tbsp olive oil
- 2 cups vegetable broth
- ⅛ tsp fresh rosemary
- ¼ tsp fresh parsley
- ¼ tsp fresh thyme
- ½ tsp sea salt

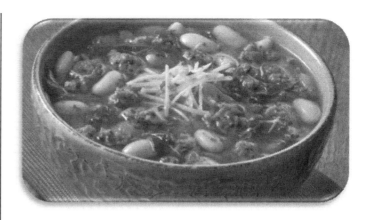

Instructions:

1. Drain the white beans, rinse, and dry.
2. Mince the garlic. Dice carrots, onions, and celery.
3. Heat olive oil in a pot. Sauté the onions for 2–3 minutes.
4. Add carrots, garlic, and celery. Sauté for another 5 minutes.
5. Add beans, vegetable broth, and all spices and herbs. Simmer it, covered, for 20–30 minutes. Serve warm.

Broccoli & Lentil Stew

Prep time: 15 minutes

Cooking time: 30 minutes

Servings: 4

Nutrients per serving:

Carbohydrates – 24 g

Fat – 6 g

Protein – 11 g

Calories – 182

Ingredients:

- 1 tbsp extra-virgin olive oil
- 1 onion, chopped
- 1 carrot, chopped
- 2 cloves garlic, minced
- 2 cups vegetable broth
- 1 cup dried green or brown lentils
- 1 tsp dried oregano
- 6 cups broccoli florets
- Salt, pepper to taste
- ½ cup pitted green olives, sliced
- ¼ cup fresh Italian parsley, chopped

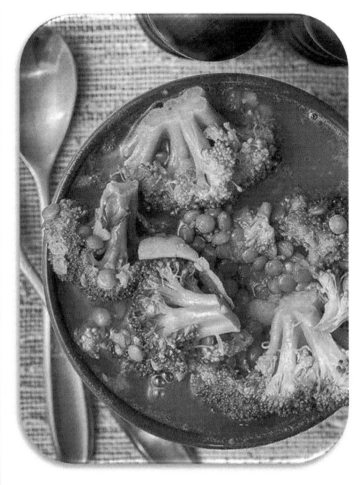

Instructions:

1. In a pot over high heat, heat the olive oil.
2. Add the onion, carrot, and garlic. Sauté for 5 minutes.
3. Add the vegetable broth, lentils, and oregano and bring to a boil. Reduce the heat to simmer. Cook the soup for 15–20 minutes.
4. Add the broccoli, cover the pot, and simmer for another 5 minutes.
5. Remove the pot from the heat and stir in the olives and parsley.
6. Pour the soup into bowls, drizzle with a little olive oil and serve.

Mango & Black Bean Stew

Prep time: 10 minutes

Cooking time: 10 minutes

Servings: 4

Nutrients per serving:

Carbohydrates – 72 g

Fat – 9 g

Protein – 20 g

Calories – 431

Ingredients:

- 2 tbsp coconut oil
- 1 onion, chopped
- 2 (15-ounce) cans black beans, drained, rinsed
- 1 tbsp chili powder
- 1 tsp salt
- ¼ tsp freshly ground black pepper
- 1 cup water
- 2 ripe mangos, sliced
- ¼ cup fresh cilantro, chopped, divided
- ¼ cup scallions, sliced, divided

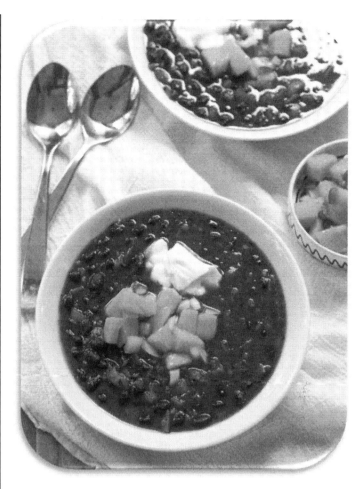

Instructions:

1. In a pot over high heat, melt the coconut oil.
2. Add the onion and sauté for 5 minutes.
3. Add the black beans, chili powder, salt, pepper, and water. Bring to a boil, then reduce the heat and simmer for 5 minutes.
4. Remove the pot from the heat; stir in the mangos just before serving. Garnish each serving with the cilantro and scallions.

Coconut Fish Stew

Prep time: 15 minutes

Cooking time: 10 minutes

Servings: 4

Nutrients per serving:

Carbohydrates – 13 g

Fat – 43 g

Protein –46 g

Calories – 80

Ingredients:

- 2 tbsp coconut oil
- 1 white onion, sliced
- 2 garlic cloves, sliced
- 2 zucchini, sliced
- 1½ pounds firm white fish fillet, cut into cubes
- 1 (4-inch) piece lemongrass, bruised
- 1 (13.5-ounce) can coconut milk
- Salt, white pepper, to taste
- ½ cup slivered scallions
- ¼ cup cilantro, chopped
- 3 tbsp lemon juice, freshly squeezed

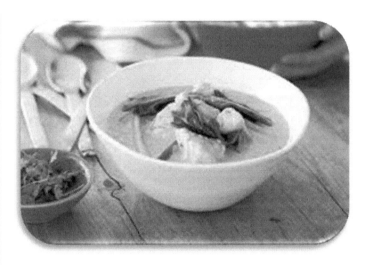

Instructions:

1. In a pot over medium heat, melt the coconut oil.
2. Add the onion, garlic, and zucchini. Sauté for 5 minutes.
3. Add the fish, lemongrass, coconut milk, salt, and white pepper to the pot. Bring to a boil, then reduce heat and simmer for 5 minutes. Remove the lemongrass.
4. Mix in the lemon juice and garnish the soup with the scallions and cilantro. Serve.

Roasted Vegetable Soup

Prep time: 30 minutes

Cooking time: 40 minutes

Servings: 6–8

Nutrients per serving:

Carbohydrates – 13 g

Fat – 17 g

Protein – 2 g

Calories – 97

Ingredients:

- 4 carrots, halved
- ½ head cauliflower, broken into florets
- 2 cups butternut squash, cubed
- 3 shallots, halved
- 3 Roma tomatoes, quartered
- 4 garlic cloves
- ½ cup extra-virgin olive oil
- Salt, pepper to taste
- 4–6 cups water or vegetable broth

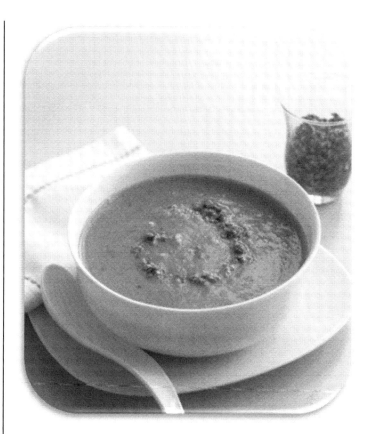

Instructions:

1. Preheat the oven to 400°F.
2. In a bowl, combine the carrots, cauliflower, butternut squash, shallots, tomatoes, and garlic. Add the olive oil, salt, and pepper and toss the vegetables to coat.
3. On a baking sheet, arrange the vegetables in a single layer. Roast the vegetables in the oven for 25 minutes.
4. Transfer the roasted vegetables to a Dutch oven over high heat. Add water or broth to cover the vegetables and bring to a boil. Reduce the heat to a simmer and cook for 10 minutes.
5. Pour the soup into a blender, and purée until smooth.

Mushrooms in Broth

Prep time: 15 minutes

Cooking time: 10 minutes

Servings: 4

Nutrients per serving:

Carbohydrates – 9 g

Fat – 5 g

Protein – 9 g

Calories – 111

Ingredients:

- 1 tbsp extra-virgin olive oil
- 1 onion, halved, sliced thin
- 3 garlic cloves, sliced
- 1 celery stalk, chopped
- 1 pound mushrooms, sliced
- Salt, pepper to taste
- 4 cups vegetable broth
- 2 tbsp fresh tarragon, chopped

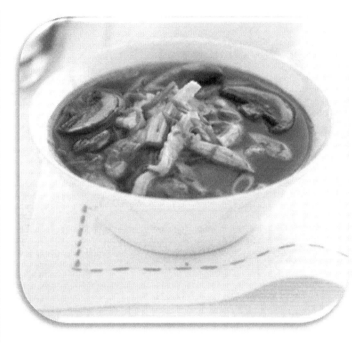

Instructions:

1. In a pot over high heat, heat the olive oil.
2. Add the onion, garlic, and celery. Sauté for 3 minutes.
3. Add the mushrooms, salt, and pepper. Sauté for 5 to 10 minutes more.
4. Add the vegetable broth and bring the soup to a boil. Reduce the heat to simmer. Cook for another 5 minutes.
5. Stir in the tarragon and serve.

Fennel, Leek & Pear Soup

Prep time: 15 minutes

Cooking time: 15 minutes

Servings: 4–6

Nutrients per serving:

Carbohydrates – 33 g

Fat – 15 g

Protein – 5 g

Calories – 267

Ingredients:

- 2 tbsp extra-virgin olive oil
- 2 leeks, sliced
- 1 fennel bulb, cut into ¼-inch-thick slices
- 2 pears, peeled, cored, and cut into ½-inch cubes
- Salt, pepper to taste
- ½ cup cashews
- 3 cups water or vegetable broth
- 2 cups packed spinach

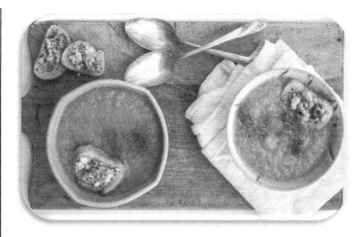

Instructions:

1. In a Dutch oven over high heat, heat the olive oil.
2. Add the leeks and fennel. Sauté for 5 minutes.
3. Add the pears, salt, and pepper. Sauté for another 3 minutes.
4. Add the cashews and water or broth and bring the soup to a boil. Reduce the heat to simmer and cook for 5 minutes, partially covered.
5. Stir in the spinach.
6. Pour the soup into a blender, and purée until smooth.

Lentil & Carrot Soup with Ginger

Prep time: 15 minutes

Cooking time: 10 minutes

Servings: 4–6

Nutrients per serving:

Carbohydrates – 28 g

Fat – 5 g

Protein – 14 g

Calories – 207

Ingredients:

- 1 tbsp coconut oil
- 2 carrots, sliced
- 1 small white onion, peeled, sliced
- 2 garlic cloves, peeled, sliced
- 1 tbsp fresh ginger, chopped
- 3 cups water or vegetable broth
- 1 (15-ounce) can lentils, drained, rinsed
- 2 tbsp fresh cilantro, chopped
- Salt, pepper to taste

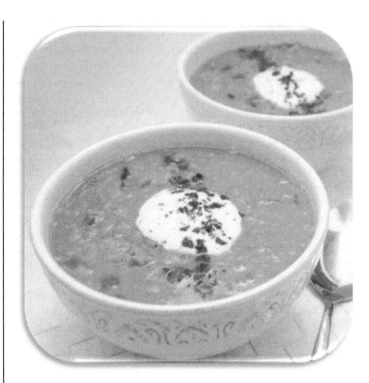

Instructions:

1. In a pot over medium-high heat, melt the coconut oil. Add the carrots, onion, garlic, and ginger. Sauté for 5 minutes.
2. Pour the water or broth into the pot and bring to a boil. Reduce the heat to simmer and cook for 5 minutes.
3. Add the lentils, cilantro, salt, and pepper. Stir well, and serve.

SALADS

Avocado & Grapefruit Salad

Prep time: 10 minutes

Cooking time: none

Servings: 2

Nutrients per serving:

Carbohydrates – 14.2 g

Fat – 19.7 g

Protein – 2.5 g

Calories – 228

Ingredients:

- 1 organic avocado
- 1 organic grapefruit
- ½ tsp dried mint
- ½ tsp sea salt

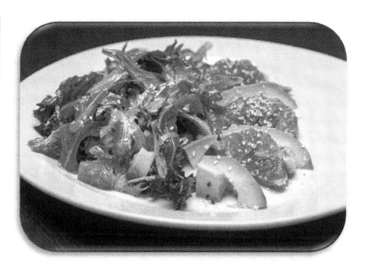

Instructions:

1. Peel grapefruit and avocado, cut into cubes.
2. Reserve avocado shells (we are using them as bowls later).
3. Gently toss avocado and grapefruit with sea salt and mint. Serve this side salad in the reserved avocado "bowls."

Super Pineapple Almond Salad

Prep time: 15 minutes

Cooking time: none

Servings: 4

Nutrients per serving:

Carbohydrates – 37 g

Fat – 13 g

Protein – 4 g

Calories – 253

Ingredients:

- 2 romaine lettuce hearts, chopped
- 1 cucumber, peeled, cut into cubes
- 2 ripe mangos, cut into cubes
- 2 scallions, sliced
- 1 large ripe avocado, cut into cubes

For the dressing:

- 8 ounces plain coconut milk yogurt
- 2 tbsp lemon juice, freshly squeezed
- 2 tbsp fresh parsley, chopped
- 1 tbsp fresh chives, snipped
- Salt, pepper to taste

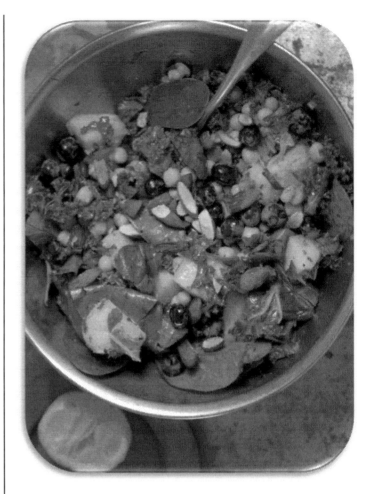

Instructions:

1. In a serving bowl, combine the romaine lettuce, cucumber, mangos, scallions, and avocado.
2. In a medium bowl, whisk together the yogurt, lemon juice, parsley, chives, salt, and pepper.
3. Pour the Creamy Coconut-Herb Dressing over the fruit and vegetables. Toss to combine.

Brussels Sprout Slaw

Prep time: 15 minutes

Cooking time: none

Servings: 4

Nutrients per serving:

Carbohydrates – 29 g

Fat – 8 g

Protein – 6 g

Calories – 189

Ingredients:

- 1 pound Brussels sprouts, sliced
- ½ red onion, sliced
- 1 apple, cored, sliced
- 1 tsp Dijon mustard
- 1 tsp salt
- 1 tbsp raw honey
- 2 tsp apple cider vinegar
- 1 cup plain coconut milk yogurt
- ½ cup chopped toasted hazelnuts
- ½ cup pomegranate seeds

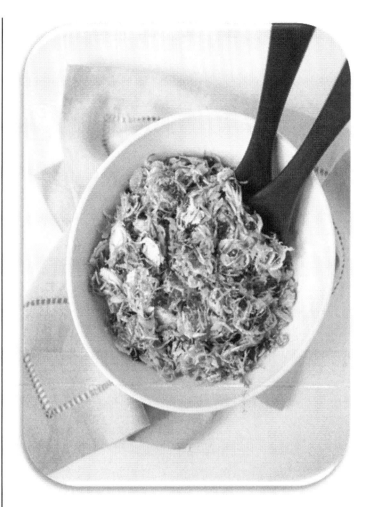

Instructions:

1. In a bowl, mix the Brussels sprouts, onion, and apple.
2. In a small bowl, whisk together the Dijon mustard, salt, honey, cider vinegar, and yogurt.
3. Add the dressing to the Brussels sprouts and toss until evenly coated.
4. Garnish the salad with the hazelnuts and pomegranate seeds.

Quinoa and Roasted Asparagus Salad

Prep time: 10 minutes

Cooking time: 15 minutes

Servings: 4

Nutrients per serving:

Carbohydrates – 24 g

Fat – 13 g

Protein – 6 g

Calories – 228

Ingredients:

- 1 bunch asparagus, trimmed
- 3 tbsp extra-virgin olive oil, divided
- 1 tsp salt, plus additional for seasoning
- 2 cups cooked quinoa, at room temperature
- ¼ red onion, chopped
- 1 tbsp apple cider vinegar
- ¼ cup fresh mint, chopped
- 1 tbsp flaxseed
- Pepper to taste

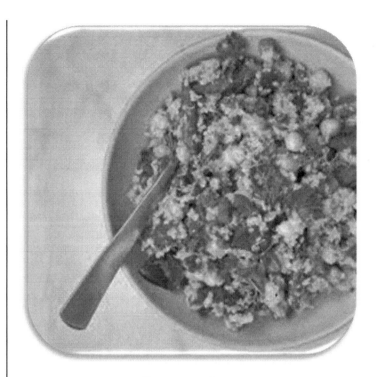

Instructions:

1. Preheat the oven to 400°F.
2. In a bowl, combine the asparagus with 1 tbsp of olive oil and 1 tsp of salt.
3. Wrap the asparagus in aluminum foil in a single layer and place the pouch on a baking sheet. Roast the asparagus in the oven for 10–15 minutes.
4. While the asparagus is roasting, mix together the quinoa, onion, vinegar, mint, flaxseed, and the remaining 2 tbsp olive oil in a bowl.
5. Once the asparagus is cool enough, slice it into pieces. Add them to the quinoa and season with salt and pepper.

White Bean & Tuna Salad

Prep time: 15 minutes

Cooking time: none

Servings: 4

Nutrients per serving:

Carbohydrates – 28 g

Fat – 19 g

Protein – 29 g

Calories – 373

Ingredients:

- 4 cups arugula
- 2 (5-ounce) cans flaked white tuna
- 1 (15-ounce) can white beans
- ½ pint cherry tomatoes halved
- ½ red onion, chopped
- ½ cup pitted kalamata olives
- ¼ cup extra-virgin olive oil
- 2 tbsp lemon juice, freshly squeezed
- Salt, pepper to taste
- 2 ounces crumbled sheep's milk or goat's milk feta cheese

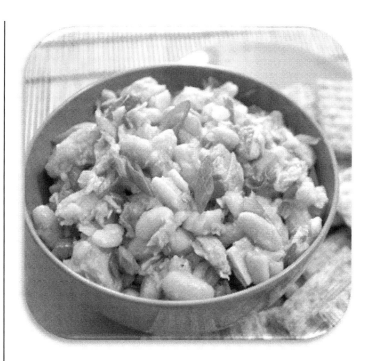

Instructions:

1. In a bowl, mix together the arugula, tuna, white beans, tomatoes, onion, olives, olive oil, and lemon juice. Season with salt and pepper.
2. Top the salad with the feta cheese.

Mango Salsa

Prep time: 15 minutes

Cooking time: none

Servings: 2

Nutrients per serving:

Carbohydrates – 10 g

Fat – 0 g

Protein – 0 g

Calories – 40

Ingredients:

- 2 cups mango, chopped
- ½ cup red onion, minced
- ¼ cup fresh cilantro, chopped
- 1 garlic clove, minced
- 1 tbsp lemon juice, freshly squeezed
- Salt to taste

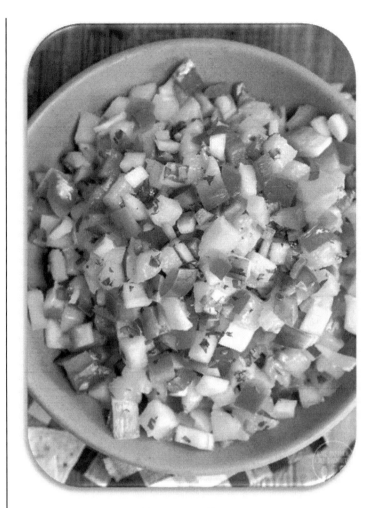

Instructions:

1. In a bowl combine all ingredients. Mix well.
2. Serve or store in an airtight container for up to one week.

Mediterranean Chopped Salad

Prep time: 15 minutes

Cooking time: none

Servings: 2

Nutrients per serving:

Carbohydrates – 15 g

Fat – 14 g

Protein – 4 g

Calories – 194

Ingredients:

- 2 cups packed spinach
- 3 large tomatoes, diced
- 1 bunch radishes, sliced thin
- 1 English cucumber, peeled and diced
- 2 scallions, sliced
- 2 garlic cloves, minced
- 1 tbsp fresh mint, chopped
- 1 tbsp fresh parsley, chopped
- 1 cup almond yogurt
- ¼ cup extra-virgin olive oil
- 3 tbsp lemon juice, freshly squeezed
- 1 tbsp apple cider vinegar
- Salt, pepper to taste
- 1 tbsp sumac

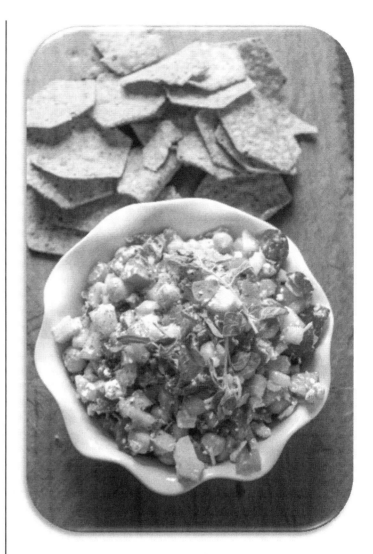

Instructions:

1. In a bowl, combine the spinach, tomatoes, radishes, cucumber, scallions, garlic, mint, parsley, yogurt, olive oil, lemon juice, cider vinegar, salt, pepper, and sumac. Toss to combine.

MAIN DISHES

Trout with Sweet-and-Sour Chard

Prep time: 15 minutes

Cooking time: 15 minutes

Servings: 4

Nutrients per serving:

Carbohydrates – 13 g

Fat – 10 g

Protein – 24 g

Calories – 231

Ingredients:

- 4 boneless trout fillets
- Salt, pepper to taste
- 1 tbsp extra-virgin olive oil
- 1 onion, chopped
- 2 garlic cloves, minced
- 2 bunches chard, sliced
- ¼ cup golden raisins
- 1 tbsp apple cider vinegar
- ½ cup vegetable broth

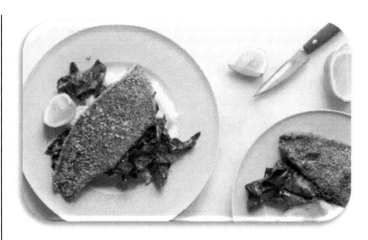

Instructions:

1. Preheat the oven to 375°F.
2. Season the trout with salt and pepper.
3. In an ovenproof pan heat the olive oil. Add the onion and garlic. Sauté for 3 minutes; add the chard and sauté for 2 minutes more.
4. Add the raisins, cider vinegar, and broth to the pan. Layer the trout fillets on top. Cover the pan and place it in the preheated oven for about 10 minutes, or until the trout is cooked through.

Pecan-Crusted Trout

Prep time: 15 minutes

Cooking time: 15 minutes

Servings: 4

Nutrients per serving:

Carbohydrates – 13 g

Fat – 59 g

Protein – 30 g

Calories – 672

Ingredients:

- Extra-virgin olive oil, for brushing
- 4 large boneless trout fillets
- Salt, pepper to taste
- 1 cup pecans, finely ground, divided
- 1 tbsp coconut oil, melted, divided
- 2 tbsp chopped fresh thyme leaves
- Lemon wedges, for garnish

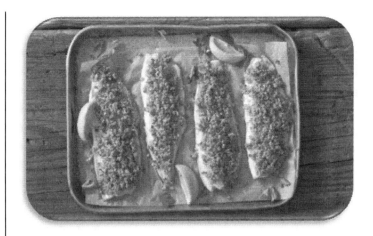

Instructions:

1. Preheat the oven to 375°F.
2. Brush a baking sheet with olive oil.
3. Place the trout fillets on the baking sheet skin-side down. Season with salt and pepper.
4. Gently press ¼ cup of ground pecans into the flesh of each fillet.
5. Drizzle the melted coconut oil over the nuts and then sprinkle the thyme over the fillets.
6. Give each fillet another sprinkle of salt and pepper.
7. Place the sheet in the oven and bake for 15 minutes. Serve warm with lemon wedges.

Sea Bass Baked with Tomatoes, Olives & Capers

Prep time: 10 minutes

Cooking time: 15 minutes

Servings: 4

Nutrients per serving:

Carbohydrates – 5 g

Fat – 12 g

Protein – 35 g

Calories – 273

Ingredients:

- 2 tbsp extra-virgin olive oil
- 4 (5-ounce) sea bass fillets
- 1 small onion, diced
- ½ cup chicken broth
- 1 cup canned diced tomatoes
- ½ cup kalamata olives, pitted, chopped
- 2 tbsp capers, drained
- 2 cups packed spinach
- 1 tsp salt
- ¼ tsp freshly ground black pepper

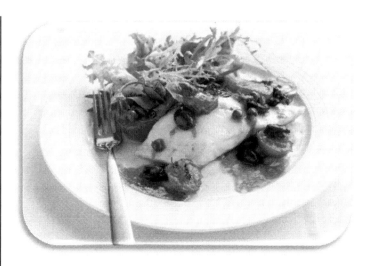

Instructions:

1. Preheat the oven to 375°F.
2. Add the olive oil to a baking dish. Place the fish fillets in the dish, turning to coat both sides with the oil.
3. Top the fish with the onion, chicken broth, tomatoes, olives, capers, spinach, salt, and pepper.
4. Cover the baking dish with aluminum foil and place it in the preheated oven. Bake for 15 minutes. Serve warm.

Swordfish with Pineapple & Cilantro

Prep time: 15 minutes

Cooking time: 20 minutes

Servings: 4

Nutrients per serving:

Carbohydrates – 7 g

Fat – 16 g

Protein – 60 g

Calories – 408

Ingredients:

- 1 tbsp coconut oil
- 2 pounds swordfish, cut into 2-inch pieces
- 1 cup fresh pineapple chunks
- ¼ cup fresh cilantro, chopped
- 2 tbsp fresh parsley, chopped
- 2 garlic cloves, minced
- 1 tbsp coconut aminos
- Salt, pepper to taste

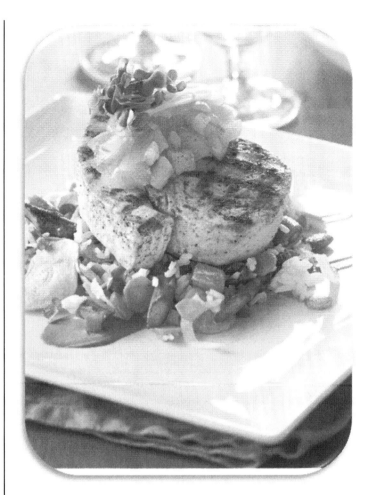

Instructions:

1. Preheat the oven to 400°F.
2. Grease a baking dish with the coconut oil.
3. Add the swordfish, pineapple, cilantro, parsley, garlic, coconut aminos, salt, and pepper to the dish. Gently mix the ingredients together.
4. Place the dish in the oven and bake for 15 to 20 minutes, or until the fish feels firm to the touch. Serve warm.

Chicken Breast with Cherry Sauce

Prep time: 10 minutes

Cooking time: 30 minutes

Servings: 4

Nutrients per serving:

Carbohydrates – 17 g

Fat – 14 g

Protein – 43 g

Calories – 379

Ingredients:

- 1 tbsp coconut oil
- 4 boneless skinless chicken breasts
- Salt, pepper to taste
- 2 scallions, sliced
- ¾ cup chicken broth
- 1 tbsp balsamic vinegar
- ½ cup dried cherries

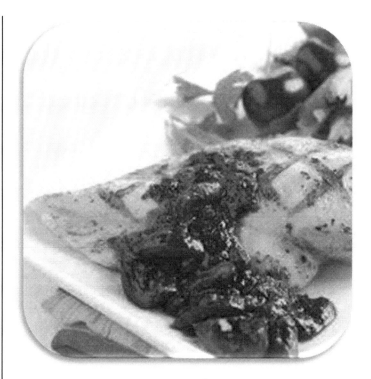

Instructions:

1. Preheat the oven to 375°F.
2. In an ovenproof skillet, melt the coconut oil.
3. Season the chicken with salt and pepper. Brown it in the pan on both sides, 3 minutes per side.
4. Add the scallions, chicken broth, balsamic vinegar, and cherries. Place the pan in the preheated oven. Bake for 20 minutes, covered. Serve warm.

Cheesy Cauliflower

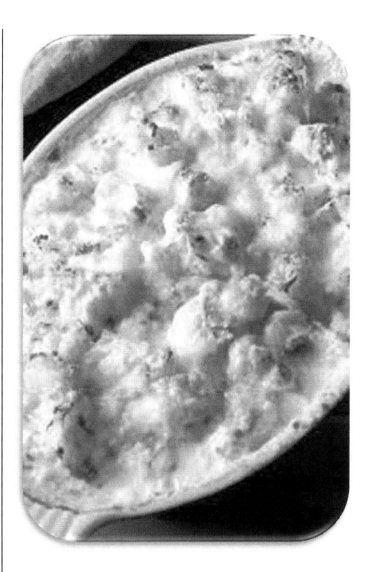

Prep time: 10 minutes

Cooking time: 50 minutes

Servings: 6

Nutrients per serving:

Carbohydrates – 11.2 g

Fat – 17.6 g

Protein – 13 g

Calories – 246

Ingredients:

- 1 medium head of cauliflower
- 1 leek, rinsed and sliced
- 17½ oz ricotta cheese
- 1 oz Parmesan cheese, grated
- 7 oz soy milk or almond milk
- ½ tsp nutmeg, ground
- 4½ oz water

Instructions:

1. Preheat the oven to 350 F.
2. Cut the cauliflower into small florets; place them in a pot.
3. Add water, cover it and steam for 5 minutes.
4. Sauté leek in 2 tbsp of olive oil.
5. Place leek and cauliflower in a baking dish.
6. Combine ricotta, ½ tsp of nutmeg and 5 oz milk together and blend till smooth.
7. Add the rest of milk. Cook till desired consistency is achieved.
8. Pour the cheese sauce over the leek and cauliflower, then sprinkle with parmesan.
9. Bake for 40 minutes. Serve.

Immune-Boosting Rice Congee

Prep time: 10 minutes

Cooking time: 1 hour 15 minutes

Servings: 2

Nutrients per serving:

Carbohydrates – 69.1 g

Fat – 3.1 g

Protein – 6.9 g

Calories – 334

Ingredients:

- 6 oz brown rice
- 64 fl oz vegetable stock or water
- ¼ tsp cold-pressed sesame oil
- 1 spring onion, sliced
- Pinch of shichimi togarashi
- Fresh ginger to taste, sliced
- Tamari to taste
- Cilantro to taste

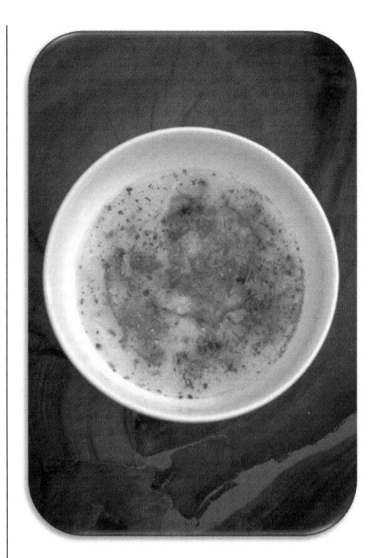

Instructions:

1. Place the rice in a pot and dry-roast it over low heat till fragrant.
2. Pour in the stock or water and bring to a boil.
3. Reduce the heat to simmer, cover it and cook for about 1 hour or till rice becomes soft.
4. Spoon it into serving bowls and garnish with shichimi togarashi, sliced ginger, cilantro, sesame oil, and tamari.

Chicken with Brown Rice & Snow Peas

Prep time: 10 minutes

Cooking time: 5 minutes

Servings: 4

Nutrients per serving:

Carbohydrates – 39 g

Fat – 7 g

Protein – 15 g

Calories – 285

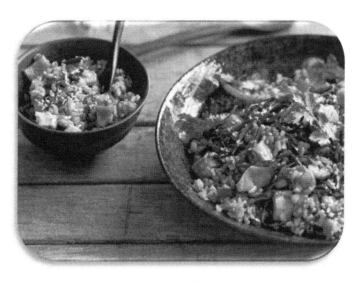

Ingredients:

- 1 tbsp coconut oil
- 2 cups brown rice, cooked
- 1 cup cooked chicken, cut into cubes
- 4 ounces snow peas, strings removed
- ½ cup chicken broth
- 1 tsp salt
- ½ tsp ginger, ground
- 1 tsp sesame seeds, toasted
- 1 tsp coconut aminos
- 2 scallions, sliced

Instructions:

1. In a pan over high heat, melt the coconut oil. Add the rice and chicken. Sauté for about 2 minutes.
2. Add the snow peas, chicken broth, salt, and ginger. Cover the pan, reduce the heat, cook for 3 minutes, or until the snow peas turn bright green.
3. Remove the pan from the heat. Stir in the sesame seeds, coconut aminos, and scallions.

Chicken Thighs with Sweet Potatoes

Prep time: 10 minutes

Cooking time: 45 minutes

Servings: 4–6

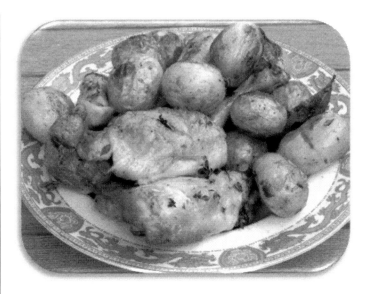

Nutrients per serving:

Carbohydrates – 22 g

Fat – 33 g

Protein – 33 g

Calories – 524

Ingredients:

- 2 tbsp extra-virgin olive oil or coconut oil
- 2 shallots, sliced thin
- 1 tsp salt
- ½ tsp cumin, ground
- ½ tsp cinnamon, ground
- ¼ tsp black pepper, freshly ground
- 1 cup chicken broth
- 6 bone-in chicken thighs
- 2 sweet potatoes, peeled and cut into ½-inch cubes

Instructions:

1. Preheat the oven to 425°F.
2. In a baking dish, stir together the oil, shallots, salt, cumin, cinnamon, pepper, and broth.
3. Add the chicken and sweet potatoes. Stir to coat with the spices.
4. Place the dish in the oven and bake for 35–45 minutes. Serve.

SIDE DISHES

Spicy Cauliflower

Prep time: 20 minutes

Cooking time: 30 minutes

Servings: 8

Nutrients per serving:

Carbohydrates – 8 g

Fat – 13 g

Protein – 3 g

Calories – 150

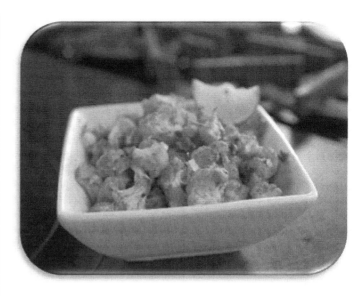

Ingredients:

- 4 tbsp extra virgin olive oil
- 1 head cauliflower, cut into florets
- 1 tsp ground cumin
- ½ tsp chili powder
- 1 tbsp curry powder
- 1 pinch cayenne pepper
- ½ tsp turmeric or cumin, ground
- 3 tbsp tomato paste
- 1½ cups vegetable stock
- ½ cup California walnuts, chopped, toasted

Instructions:

1. In the skillet over medium heat, heat 3 tbsp olive oil; add cauliflower florets. Cook for 15–20 minutes.
2. Remove the cauliflower florets from pan and keep aside.
3. Return the pan to heat; add remaining olive oil. Add curry powder, chili powder, cayenne pepper, and ground turmeric (or cumin); stir for about 30 seconds.
4. Add tomato paste and vegetable stock and stir well to blend.
5. Return cauliflower florets to pan; stir for 2–3 minutes.
6. Add toasted walnuts, combine well, and serve.

Strawberry Avocado Tostada

Prep time: 10 minutes

Cooking time: 10 minutes

Servings: 6

Nutrients per serving:

Carbohydrates – 30 g

Fat – 14 g

Protein – 5 g

Calories – 25

Ingredients:

- 2½ cups fresh California strawberries, quartered
- 1 lb avocados, seeded, diced
- ½ lb jicama, peeled, diced
- 1 tsp jalapeño peppers, minced
- 2 tbsp lime juice
- ½ cup cilantro, chopped
- 6 (6-inch) yellow corn tortillas
- 6 tbsp queso fresco, crumbled
- Chili powder
- 6 cilantro sprigs
- 1 lime, cut into 6 wedges

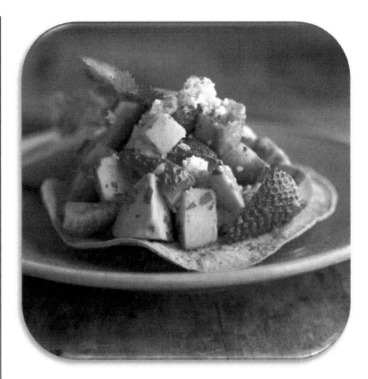

Instructions:

1. Heat the oven at 400°F.
2. In a bowl, mix strawberries, cilantro, jicama, lime juice, and peppers together. Add avocados; fold them together gently.
3. Arrange corn tortillas on the oven rack. Toast them for 10 minutes.
4. Put strawberry mixture in the center of each tortilla. Sprinkle all tostadas with 1 tbsp of queso fresco and chili powder. Garnish them with cilantro or a lime wedge.

Rosemary Squash

Prep time: 20 minutes
Cooking time: 40 minutes
Servings: 8

Nutrients per serving:

Carbohydrates – 17.8 g

Fat – 5.2 g

Protein – 1.4 g

Calories – 116.2

Ingredients:

- 2 winter squash, such as acorn or spaghetti
- 2 sweet potatoes, unpeeled
- 3 tbsp extra-virgin olive oil
- 2 tsp rosemary
- ½ tsp sea salt or to taste
- ¼ tsp pepper or to taste

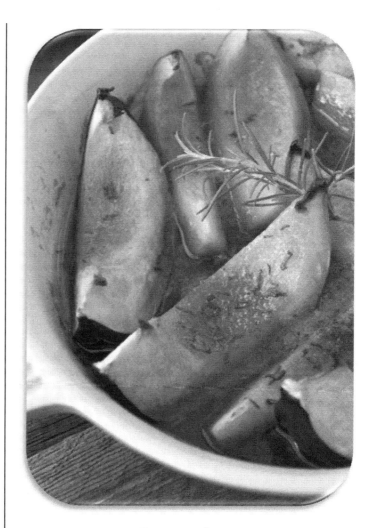

Instructions:

1. Seed and chop the squash into 3/4-inch chunks, removing the shell.
2. Chop the sweet potatoes into 3/4-inch chunks.
3. Mix the sweet potatoes and squash, drizzle with olive oil and add seasonings.
4. Cover and bake for about 40 minutes. Stir occasionally during the baking process.

Scrumptious Green Beans

Prep time: 10 minutes

Cooking time: 30 minutes

Servings: 6

Nutrients per serving:

Carbohydrates – 6.5 g

Fat – 4.7 g

Protein – 1.5 g

Calories – 68.6

Ingredients:

- 2 tbsp olive oil
- ½ tsp black or yellow mustard seeds, available in the bulk herb section of most health food stores
- ½-inch cube of peeled ginger, julienned thin
- ¼ cup water
- 1 pound green beans, washed and trimmed
- ½ tsp ground cumin
- ¼ tsp turmeric
- 1 tsp sea salt
- 2 tbsp minced fresh cilantro
- Juice of 1 lemon

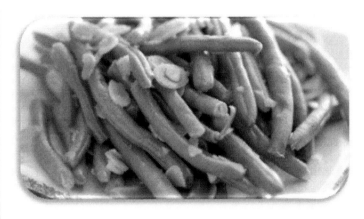

Instructions:

1. Sauté mustard seeds and ginger in olive oil over moderate heat until mustard seeds begin to pop.
2. Add the beans and stir-fry over medium heat for about 5 minutes.
3. Add the water, cover tightly, and simmer for 5 minutes.
4. Remove the lid when most of the water has evaporated. Add all remaining ingredients except lemon juice, and continue cooking until the beans are warm but still slightly crisp.
5. Add the lemon juice just before serving. Serve warm.

Simple & Delectable Beets

Prep time: 10 minutes

Cooking time: 30 minutes

Servings: 4

Nutrients per serving:

Carbohydrates – 6 g

Fat – 0.1 g

Protein – 1 g

Calories – 26.8 g

Ingredients:

- 3 beets, peeled and steamed until tender, but still slightly crunchy
- 1 tsp lemon juice
- 1 tsp honey (optional)
- Sea salt and pepper to taste

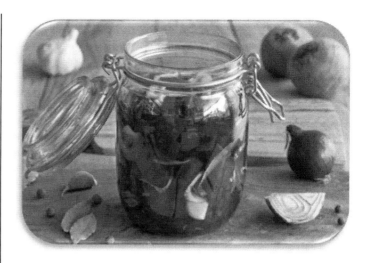

Instructions:

1. Steam beets and set aside to cool slightly.
2. Mix lemon juice and honey together over low heat in a 2-quart saucepan until well blended.
3. Turn off heat. Slice beets, and add them to the pan. Mix gently.
4. Add sea salt, pepper to taste, and serve immediately.
5. If you are omitting the honey, just sprinkle the beets with lemon juice, sea salt, and pepper and serve.

Cauliflower Purée

Prep time: 15 minutes

Cooking time: 10 minutes

Servings: 4

Nutrients per serving:

Carbohydrates – 6 g

Fat – 11 g

Protein – 2 g

Calories – 117 g

Ingredients:

- 1 head cauliflower, broken into florets
- 1 garlic clove
- Salt, pepper, to taste
- ½ cup coconut milk
- 1 tbsp extra-virgin olive oil

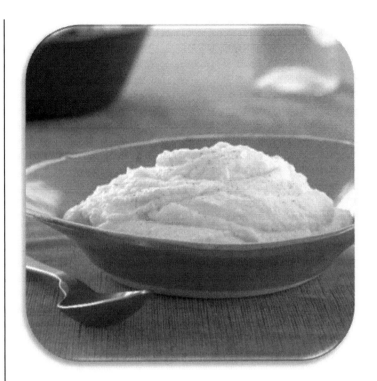

Instructions:

1. Bring a pot of water to a boil. Add the cauliflower, garlic clove, and 1 tsp of salt. Boil for 5 minutes.
2. Drain the cauliflower with the garlic clove and transfer to a large bowl. Mash with a potato masher.
3. Add the remaining 1 tsp salt, the pepper, and coconut milk to the mash. Stir to combine.
4. Place the purée in a serving bowl and drizzle with olive oil.

Green Beans with Crispy Shallots

Prep time: 15 minutes

Cooking time: 10 minutes

Servings: 4

Nutrients per serving:

Carbohydrates – 9 g

Fat – 13 g

Protein – 2 g

Calories – 146 g

Ingredients:

- 1 tsp sea salt, plus additional for seasoning
- 1 pound green beans, trimmed
- ¼ cup extra-virgin olive oil
- 1 large shallot, sliced thin
- 1 tbsp chopped fresh tarragon
- Freshly ground black pepper

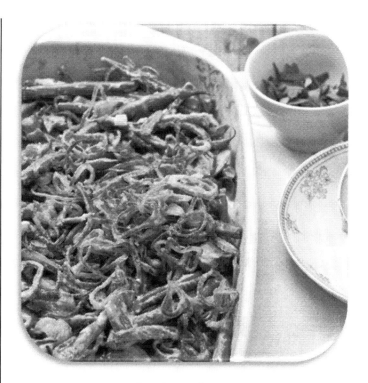

Instructions:

1. Bring a pot of water to a boil.
2. Add 1 tsp sea salt to the boiling water and add the beans to the pot. Cook for 5 minutes.
3. Drain the beans and place them in a serving dish.
4. In a small pan over medium heat, heat the olive oil. Once the oil is hot, add the shallots. Cook for 1–2 minutes.
5. Spoon the shallots over the green beans. Sprinkle with the tarragon and season with sea salt and pepper.

DESSERTS

Banana-Cocoa Ice

Prep time: 10 minutes

Cooking time: none

Servings: 6

Nutrients per serving:

Carbohydrates – 30 g

Fat – 0.7 g

Protein – 1.4 g

Calories – 118.1 g

Ingredients:

- 4 extremely ripe bananas
- 2 tbsp cocoa powder, unsweetened
- 2 tbsp maple syrup
- 1 tsp vanilla extract

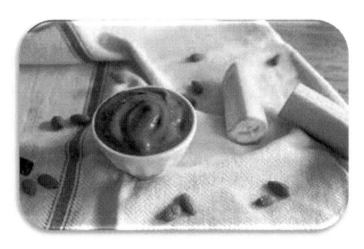

Instructions:

1. Peel bananas; place them in a food processor or blender along with cocoa powder.
2. Add maple syrup and vanilla extract.
3. Blend until smooth. Pour it into small bowls or custard cups and place in the freezer until frozen.

Melon with Berry-Yogurt Sauce

Prep time: 15 minutes

Cooking time: none

Servings: 6

Nutrients per serving:

Carbohydrates – 11 g

Fat – 4 g

Protein – 1 g

Calories – 76 g

Ingredients:

- 1 cantaloupe, peeled, sliced
- 1 pint fresh raspberries
- ½ tsp vanilla extract
- 1 cup plain coconut milk or almond milk yogurt
- ½ cup toasted coconut

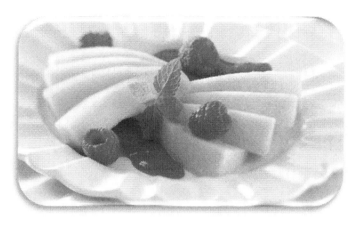

Instructions:

1. Place the melon slices on a serving plate.
2. In a bowl, mash the berries with the vanilla. Add the yogurt and stir until just mixed.
3. Spoon the berry-yogurt mixture over the melon slices and sprinkle with the coconut.

Cherry "Ice Cream"

Prep time: 10 minutes

Cooking time: none

Servings: 4-6

Nutrients per serving:

Carbohydrates – 14 g

Fat – 2 g

Protein – 1 g

Calories – 82 g

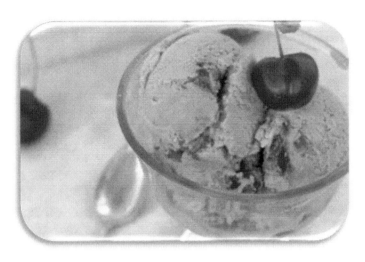

Ingredients:

- 1 (10-ounce) package frozen unsweetened cherries
- 3 cups unsweetened almond milk
- 1 tsp vanilla extract
- ½ tsp almond extract

Instructions:

1. In a blender, combine the cherries, almond milk, vanilla extract, and almond extract. Process until smooth.
2. Pour the mixture into a container with an airtight lid. Freeze before serving.

Chocolate-Avocado Mousse with Sea Salt

Prep time: 10 minutes

Cooking time: 5 minutes

Servings: 4–6

Nutrients per serving:

Carbohydrates – 56 g

Fat – 47 g

Protein – 7 g

Calories – 653 g

Ingredients:

- 8 ounces bittersweet chocolate, chopped
- ¼ cup coconut milk
- 2 tbsp coconut oil
- 2 ripe avocados
- ¼ cup raw honey or maple syrup
- Sea salt to taste

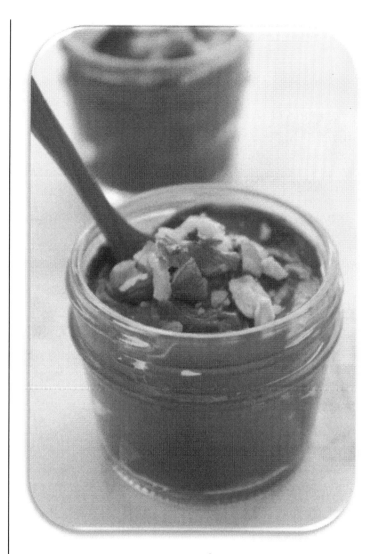

Instructions:

1. In a saucepan, combine the chocolate, coconut milk, and coconut oil. Cook for 2–3 minutes, stirring constantly.
2. In a food processor, combine the avocado and honey. Add the melted chocolate and process until smooth.
3. Put the mousse into serving bowls and top each with a sprinkle of sea salt. Chill for 30 minutes before serving.

Chocolate-Cherry Clusters

Prep time: 15 minutes

Cooking time: none

Servings: 10

Nutrients per serving:

Carbohydrates – 18 g

Fat – 13 g

Protein – 4 g

Calories – 198 g

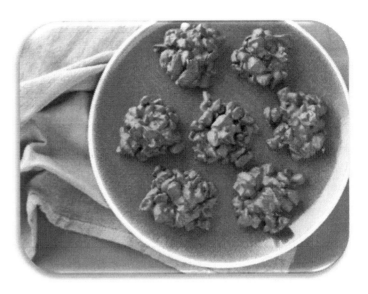

Ingredients:

- 1 cup dark chocolate, chopped
- 1 tbsp coconut oil
- 1 cup salted almonds, roasted
- ½ cup dried cherries

Instructions:

1. Line a baking sheet with wax paper.
2. Over a double boiler, stir together the chocolate and coconut oil.
3. Remove the boiler from the heat and stir in the almonds and cherries.
4. By spoonfuls, drop clusters onto the wax paper. Refrigerate until hardened.
5. Transfer to an airtight container and refrigerate.

Baked Red Apples

Prep time: 5 minutes

Cooking time: 1 hour

Servings: 1

Nutrients per serving:

Carbohydrates – 27.5 g

Fat – 0.3 g

Protein – 0.5 g

Calories – 104.3 g

Ingredients:

- 1 apple (Fuji, Braeburn,or Gala)
- 1 tsp maple syrup
- Dash of cinnamon
- 10 raisins
- Fresh lemon juice to taste
- 1 tsp filtered water

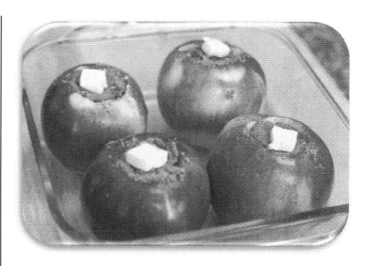

Instructions:

1. Preheat oven to 375° F.
2. Core apple. Peel skin off the top third of apple and place in a baking dish. Drizzle maple syrup, cinnamon, and raisins over apple.
3. Squeeze lemon juice on top and add 1 tsp of water to the baking dish.
4. Bake uncovered for about 1 hour, and serve warm.

Coconut Vanilla "Ice Cream"

Prep time: 30 minutes

Cooking time: none

Servings: 6

Nutrients per serving:

Carbohydrates – 17.6 g

Fat – 14.2 g

Protein – 2.8 g

Calories – 201.4 g

Ingredients:

- 1 13.5-ounce can coconut milk
- 1¼ cup vanilla soy milk
- ¼ cup honey
- 1 tbsp vanilla extract

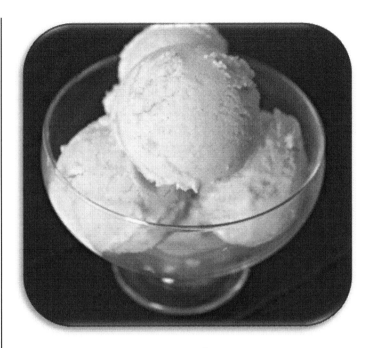

Instructions:

1. Combine all ingredients in a medium-sized bowl; mix well until honey is dissolved.
2. Turn ice cream maker on and pour mixture in.
3. Let ice cream maker operate for 30 minutes. Serve immediately.

Mochi with Yogurt

Prep time: 5 minutes

Cooking time: 16 minutes

Servings: 4

Nutrients per serving:

Carbohydrates – 82.4 g

Fat – 1.4 g

Protein – 5.9 g

Calories – 367.6 g

Ingredients:

- 1 12.5-ounce package mochi (can be found in the refrigerated section of a health-food store)
- 1 cup plain soy milk yogurt
- 1 cup blueberries
- ½ cup pure maple syrup

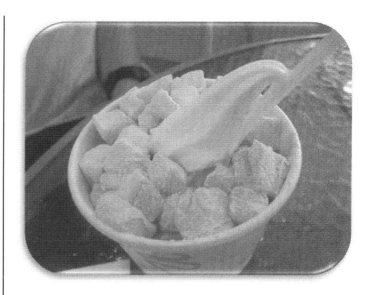

Instructions:

1. Preheat oven to 350° F.
2. Cut mochi patty into 12 pieces and arrange on lightly greased baking pan. Bake until they begin to puff up and fill with air, about 12–16 minutes. Remove from oven. Top with yogurt and blueberries, and drizzle with maple syrup. Serve immediately.

SMOOTHIES & DRINKS

Inflammation-Soothing Smoothie

Prep time: 10 minutes

Cooking time: none

Servings: 1

Nutrients per serving:

Carbohydrates – 37 g

Fat – 1 g

Protein – 4 g

Calories – 147

Ingredients:

- 1 pear, peeled, seeded, cored, quartered
- ½ fennel bulb
- 1 thin slice fresh ginger
- 1 cup spinach, packed
- ½ cucumber, peeled
- ½ cup water

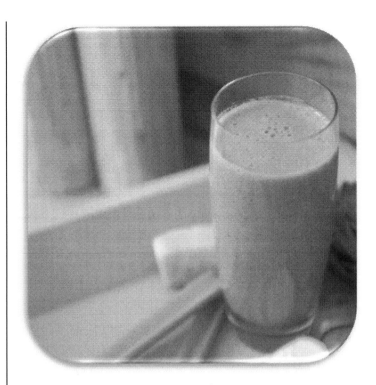

Instructions:

1. In a blender, combine the pear, fennel, ginger, spinach, cucumber, and water. Blend until smooth.

Cherry Smoothie

Prep time: 10 minutes

Cooking time: none

Servings: 1

Nutrients per serving:

Carbohydrates – 52 g

Fat – 2 g

Protein – 3 g

Calories – 266

Ingredients:

- 1 cup frozen unsweetened pitted cherries
- ¼ cup raspberries
- ¾ cup coconut water
- 1 tbsp raw honey or maple syrup
- 1 tsp chia seeds
- 1 tsp hemp seeds
- Drop vanilla extract

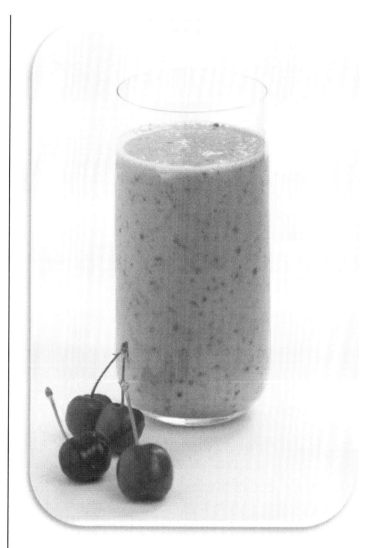

Instructions:

1. In a blender, combine the cherries, raspberries, coconut water, honey, chia seeds and hemp seeds.
2. Add vanilla and blend until smooth.

Eat-Your-Vegetables Smoothie

Prep time: 10 minutes

Cooking time: none

Servings: 1

Nutrients per serving:

Carbohydrates – 24 g

Fat – 1 g

Protein – 3 g

Calories – 140

Ingredients:

- 1 carrot, trimmed
- 1 small beet, peeled, scrubbed, quartered
- 1 celery stalk
- ½ cup fresh raspberries
- 1 cup coconut water
- 1 tsp balsamic vinegar

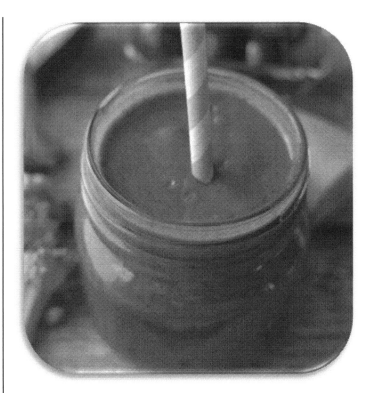

Instructions:

1. In a blender, combine the carrot, beet, celery, raspberries, coconut water, and balsamic vinegar. Blend until smooth.

Green Apple Smoothie

Prep time: 10 minutes

Cooking time: none

Servings: 1

Nutrients per serving:

Carbohydrates – 41 g

Fat – 1 g

Protein – 2 g

Calories – 176

Ingredients:

- ½ cup coconut water
- 1 green apple, peeled, cored, seeded, quartered
- 1 cup spinach
- ¼ lemon, seeded
- ½ cucumber, peeled, seeded
- 2 tsp raw honey

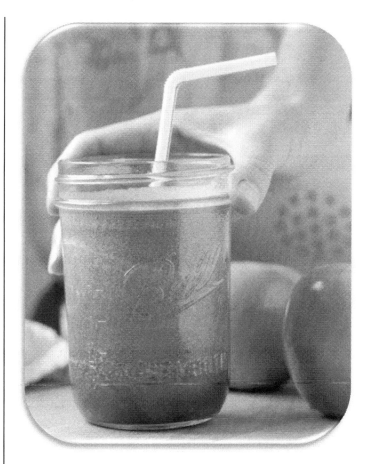

Instructions:

1. In a blender, combine the coconut water, apple, spinach, lemon, cucumber, and honey. Blend until smooth.

One-for-All Smoothie

Prep time: 10 minutes

Cooking time: none

Servings: 1

Nutrients per serving:

Carbohydrates – 27 g

Fat – 5 g

Protein – 2 g

Calories – 152

Ingredients:

- 1 cup packed spinach
- ½ cup fresh blueberries
- ½ banana
- 1 cup coconut milk
- ½ tsp vanilla extract

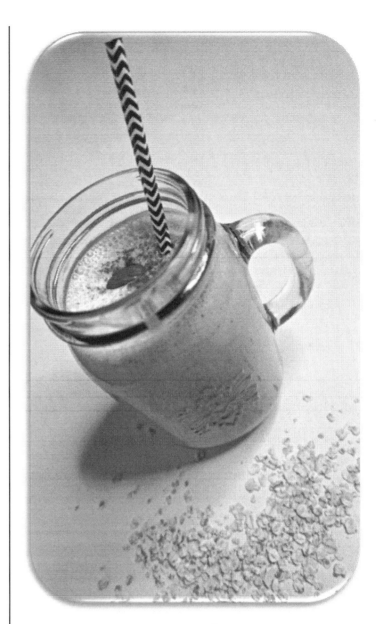

Instructions:

1. In a blender, combine the spinach, blueberries, banana, coconut milk, and vanilla. Blend until smooth.

Mango-Thyme Smoothie

Prep time: 10 minutes

Cooking time: none

Servings: 1

Nutrients per serving:

Carbohydrates – 65 g

Fat – 4 g

Protein – 3 g

Calories – 274

Ingredients:

- 1 cup mango chunks
- ½ cup white, seedless grapes
- ¼ fennel bulb
- ½ cup unsweetened almond milk
- ½ tsp fresh thyme leaves
- Salt, pepper to taste

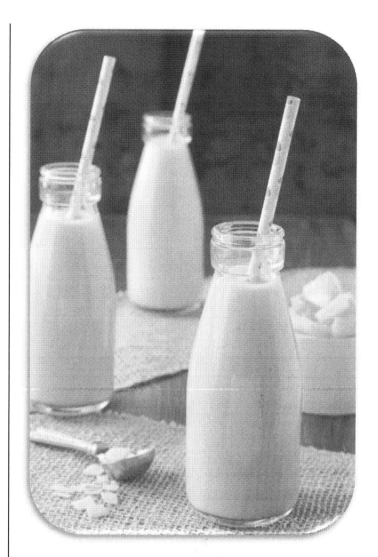

Instructions:

1. In a blender, combine the mango, grapes, fennel, almond milk, thyme leaves, sea salt, and pepper. Blend until smooth.

Protein Powerhouse Smoothie

Prep time: 10 minutes

Cooking time: none

Servings: 1

Nutrients per serving:

Carbohydrates – 47 g

Fat – 32 g

Protein – 13 g

Calories – 500

Ingredients:

- 1 cup packed kale leaves
- ¼ avocado
- 1 cup fresh grapes, seedless
- 1 tbsp hemp seed
- 2 mint leaves
- 1 cup coconut milk

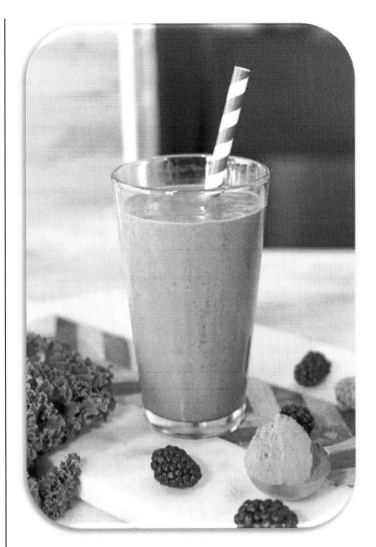

Instructions:

1. In a blender, combine the kale, avocado, grapes, hemp seed, mint leaves, and coconut milk. Blend until smooth.

Energizing Pineapple Breakfast Smoothie

Prep time: 10 minutes

Cooking time: none

Servings: 1

Nutrients per serving:

Carbohydrates – 64.4 g

Fat – 3.9 g

Protein – 27.5 g

Calories – 379

Ingredients:

- 1 cup herbal tea, brewed and then cooled
- 1 cup pineapple chunks, frozen
- ½ cup mango chunks, frozen
- ½ banana, peeled
- ½ inch fresh ginger, peeled, cut
- 2 cups kale
- 2/3 cup cucumber, peeled, diced
- 3 mint leaves, chopped
- 1 tbsp chia seeds
- ¼ tsp ground turmeric
- 1 scoop protein powder
- 4–5 ice cubes

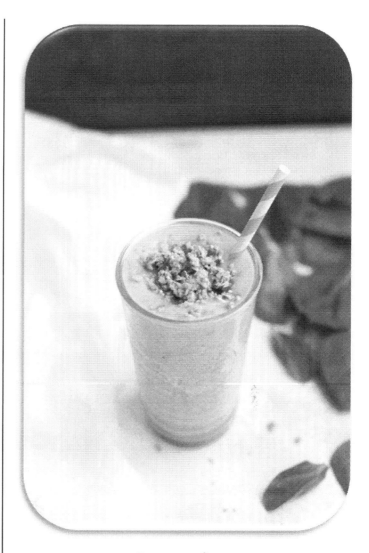

Instructions:

1. Except for chia seeds, combine all the other ingredients in a high-speed blender and blend.
2. Add chia seeds to the final stage of the blending process so that they do not stick to blender container.

Recipe Index

A
Avocado & Grapefruit Salad 45
Avocado and Egg Toast............................. 21

B
Baked Red Apples 73
Banana-Cocoa Ice 68
Broccoli & Lentil Stew............................... 38
Brussels Sprout Slaw 47
Buckwheat Crêpes with Berries 27

C
Cauliflower Purée...................................... 66
Cheesy Cauliflower.................................... 57
Cherry Ice Cream 70
Cherry Smoothie 77
Chia Breakfast Pudding 23
Chicken Breast with Cherry Sauce............. 56
Chicken Thighs with Sweet Potatoes 60
Chicken with Brown Rice & Snow Peas 59
Chocolate-Avocado Mousse with Sea Salt.. 71
Chocolate-Cherry Clusters........................ 72
Coconut Fish Stew 40
Coconut Rice with Berries 24
Coconut Vanilla "Ice Cream" 74
Cucumber-Yogurt Dip................................ 29

E
Eat-Your-Vegetables Smoothie 78
Energizing Pineapple Breakfast Smoothie 83

F
Fennel, Leek & Pear Soup......................... 43

G
Green Apple Smoothie 79
Green Beans with Crispy Shallots.............. 67

I
Immune-Boosting Rice Congee 58
Inflammation-Soothing Smoothie............. 76

L
Lemony Chia Quinoa Bowl 22
Lentil & Carrot Soup with Ginger.............. 44

M
Mango & Black Bean Stew 39
Mango Salsa 50
Mango-Thyme Smoothie 81
Mashed Avocado with Jicama Slices 30
Mediterranean Chopped Salad 51
Melon with Berry-Yogurt Sauce................. 69
Mini Snack Muffins.................................... 34
Mochi with Yogurt......................................75
Mushroom 28
Mushrooms in Broth.................................. 42

O
One-for-All Smoothie................................ 80
Oven-Roasted Parsnips.............................. 36
Overnight Muesli....................................... 25

P
Pecan-Crusted Trout.................................. 53
Plantain Fries with Garlic & Rosemary 35
Protein Powerhouse Smoothie................... 82

Q
Quinoa and Roasted Asparagus Salad 48

R
Roasted Vegetable Soup.............................41
Rosemary Squash 63

S
Scrumptious Green Beans.......................... 64
Sea Bass Baked with Tomatoes, Olives & Capers 54
Simple & Delectable Beets 65
Smoked Trout & Mango Wraps 31
Smoked Turkey–Wrapped Zucchini Sticks 32
Spicy Cauliflower.......................................61
Spicy Quinoa 26
Strawberry Avocado Tostada 62
Super Pineapple Almonds Salad................ 46
Sweet Potato Chips.................................... 33
Swordfish with Pineapple & Cilantro 55

T
Trout with Sweet-and-Sour Chard............. 52
Tuscan White Beans Stew 37

W
White Bean and Tuna Salad....................... 49

Conversion Tables

VOLUME EQUIVALENTS (LIQUID)

US STANDARD	US STANDARD (OUNCES)	METRIC
2 tablespoons	1 fl. oz.	30 mL
¼ cup	2 fl. oz.	60 mL
½ cup	4 fl. oz.	120 mL
1 cup	8 fl. oz.	240 mL
1½ cups	12 fl. oz.	355 mL
2 cups or 1 pint	16 fl. oz.	475 mL
4 cups or 1 quart	32 fl. oz.	1 L
1 gallon	128 fl. oz.	4 L

OVEN TEMPERATURES

FAHRENHEIT (°F)	CELSIUS (°C) APPROXIMATE
250 °F	120 °C
300 °F	150 °C
325 °F	165 °C
350 °F	180 °C
375 °F	190 °C
400 °F	200 °C
425 °F	220 °C
450 °F	230 °C

VOLUME EQUIVALENTS (LIQUID)

US STANDARD	METRIC (APPROXIMATE)
1/8 teaspoon	0.5 mL
¼ teaspoon	1 mL
½ teaspoon	2 mL
2/3 teaspoon	4 mL
1 teaspoon	5 mL
1 tablespoon	15 mL
¼ cup	59 mL
1/3 cup	79 mL
½ cup	118 mL
2/3 cup	156 mL
¾ cup	177 mL
1 cup	235 mL
2 cups or 1 pint	475 mL
3 cups	700 mL
4 cups or 1 quart	1 L
½ gallon	2 L
1 gallon	4 L

WEIGHT EQUIVALENTS

US STANDARD	METRIC (APPROXIMATE)
½ ounce	15 g
1 ounce	30 g
2 ounces	60 g
4 ounces	115 g
8 ounces	225 g
12 ounces	340 g
16 ounces or 1 pound	455 g

Other Books by Emma Green

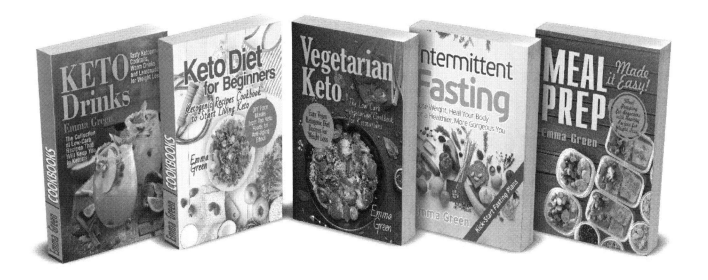

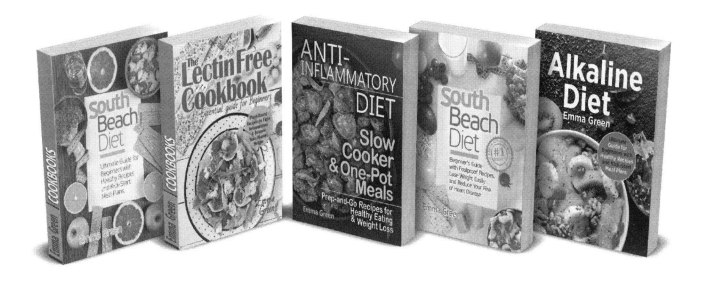

Emma Green's page on Amazon
https://goo.gl/7yn2fR